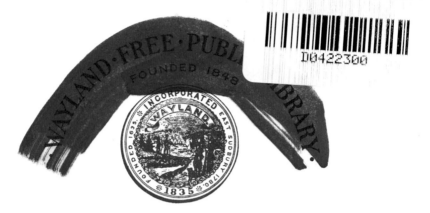

Fitness
after
50

Fitness
after
50

Herbert A. deVries, Ph.D.
with
Dianne Hales

CHARLES SCRIBNER'S SONS NEW YORK

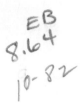
The material in this book first appeared in different form in Vigor Regained
by Herbert deVries (New York: Prentice-Hall, 1974)

Copyright © 1974, 1982 Herbert A. deVries

Library of Congress Cataloging in Publication Data

DeVries, Herbert A.
   · Fitness after 50.

Includes index.
1. Physical fitness for the aged. 2. Exercise
for the aged. 3. Middle age—Health and hygiene.
I. Hales, Dianne R., 1950–   II. Title.
III. Title: Fitness after fifty.
RA781.D48   613.7'1'0880565   82-641
   ISBN 0-684-17485-5   AACR2

1 3 5 7 9 11 13 15 17 19   F/C   20 18 16 14 12 10 8 6 4 2

Printed in the United States of America.

Contents

Part I

AGING AND FITNESS

1

It's Never Too Late to Be Fit

John is 63 and worried. Last month his neighbor suffered a heart attack. Several of his colleagues at work have had problems with high blood pressure and heart disease. Could he lessen his own risk of heart troubles?

For decades Martha, 59, has been fighting fat. She's nibbled on celery sticks and grapefruit halves—and finally succumbed to hunger pangs and binges on cake and chocolate. She's huffed and puffed through dozens of exercise programs—only to quit because of aching muscles. Could she lose weight and keep it off without starvation or strain?

The house in Florida is Harry and Mabel's retirement dream come true. But they haven't settled cozily into their new life. Both are anxious and edgy, snapping at each other over trivial irritations. And they've lost the vitality that once made them the life of every party. By 7:00 P.M. they're so pooped that they snooze through the evening news. Could they feel less tense and more energetic?

John and Martha and Harry and Mabel are not unlike many of the millions of Americans over 50: They belong to the fastest growing segment of our population. They have more options, more resources, and more rights than any generation before them. They can expect to live longer than their parents and grandparents. Yet the promise of their golden years is tarnished by a host of problems, some minor and episodic, and some serious and chronic: headaches, insomnia, back troubles, constant fatigue, tension, overweight, muscles that ache and throb, blood pressure that's ominously high. They may not be ill, yet they're not quite well. Ask them what they think the problem is and they're likely to shrug it off as "something you've got to expect when you get to this age."

But are these problems and pains truly inevitable? Must we dwindle from maturity into an old age of compromise and complaint? Does living longer have to mean living less fully? The answer is no. We *can* lessen the risk of heart disease, keep trim, soothe fraying nerves, and boost energy. But before we can delay or stop the symptoms of aging, we have to understand what happens to our bodies as we age, and why.

THE AGING BODY

The time from the late teens to age 30 is the body's finest era. Lung capacity is greatest then. Grip strength is firmest. Motor responses are quickest, and physical endurance is longest. The decline from these peak levels is slow. Aging is not something that happens only in old age; it begins decades before we notice its effects.

With each year after we reach maturity, the heart's ability to pump blood declines about 1 percent. A lining of fatty substances coats the arteries; by middle age the channels in our blood vessels are 29 percent narrower than they were in youth. Blood pressure rises, and circulation slows. In a person of 60, blood flows from arm to thigh at a rate 30 to 60 percent slower than in a 25-year-old. Strength diminishes very slowly. By age 60 men have lost only 10 to 20 percent of their maximum power; women have lost somewhat more. But the amount of oxygen the body can use—the best measure of our ability to do work—declines more rapidly. By age 75 a man's capacity is less than half that at age 17; a woman in her sixties has a maximum work capacity 29 percent lower than she had in her twenties.

As nerve cells age, reaction time and movement speed slow. Our basal metabolism, the fundamental chemical process of living, uses less energy (and fewer calories) because the aging body, with fewer cells, demands less upkeep. Each decade after age 25 we lose 3 to 5 percent of our muscle mass, and that mass is often replaced by fatty tissue. Our bones lose minerals and become softer and shorter. Women become particularly vulnerable to falls and fractures. After age 30 both sexes shrink about half an inch in total height with each decade.

IS TIME THE VILLAIN?

These are changes that *accompany* aging. There is no solid evidence that they cause or are caused by it. Gerontologists, scientists who specialize in the study of aging, believe that a combination of factors can precipitate these changes, including the passage of time, unrecognized illnesses that increase and worsen with age, and the sedentary life-style of older people. Aging, as one doctor puts it, "is not a simple slope which everyone slides down at the same speed; it is a flight of irregular stairs down which some journey more quickly than others."

Many people age more rapidly than they need to, not because of what they do, but because of what they don't do. Inactivity can make people of any age old before their time. Several years ago, researchers at the University of Southern California demonstrated this fact by confining healthy young college men to bed for two to three weeks. The volunteers in "Operation Sacktime" lost energy and strength. They couldn't perform strenuous activities; their hearts, lungs, muscles, and circulation became less efficient. After just a short period of inactivity, their young bodies acted and reacted as if they were decades older.

If just a few weeks without physical exertion can undermine fitness temporarily, decades of the no-sweat, effort-free, push-bottom American life-style can do far worse. Thanks to medical advances, ours is the first civilization in history to be spared the infectious diseases that once killed millions in their prime. We live twenty-three years longer than Americans did at the turn of the century. But we don't survive simply to die "of natural causes"; all too often, we self-destruct. The killers and cripplers of our society are the degenerative diseases, such as heart attacks, hypertension, strokes, respiratory problems, arthritis, and connective tissue disorders. We rust out long before we wear out, largely because we fail to put our bodies to proper use.

In the past fifty to seventy-five years, physical activity has become the exception rather than the rule, both at home and on the job. We drive where others once walked. We flick a switch and machines do our hauling, lifting, pushing, and pulling for us. On weekends we get our exercise vicariously by watching professional athletes on television. What we do—and overdo—is as harmful as what we don't do. We eat too much, drink too much, and smoke too much, and we ignore a disturbing fact of life: that what we do and don't do every day affects how long and how well we'll live. In a now-classic study of the impact of daily habits on health, California researchers surveyed almost seven thousand persons about their smoking, drinking, hours of sleep, breakfast eating, meal regularity, weight, and physical activity. Men who had good habits in six or seven of these areas lived eleven years longer than those with fewer than four; the difference in life expectancy for women with and without good habits was seven years.

Of all healthful habits, exercise may be the most important. We were designed to be active. The unexercised body, even if free from the symptoms of illness, is not at its full potential—not in a state of positive well-being. This state of mind and body meets the same definition that the President's Council on Physical Fitness uses to define optimum health: "a reflection of your ability to work with vigorous pleasure, without undue fatigue, with energy left for enjoying hobbies and recreational activities and for meeting unseen emergencies . . . it relates to how you feel mentally as well as physically."

The quest for fitness has pulled more than 17 million Americans out of their armchairs and into running shoes. The president's fitness council describes the current trend as "the first peacetime exercise boom in history and the first ever to include women and older people." In one recent marathon in New York City, 423 runners were between the ages of 50 and 60; 41 competitors were over 60. In almost every marathon or endurance race, the oldest runners are likely to get as many headlines as the fastest ones.

Most Americans over 50, however, are still right where they always were—sitting back and watching others jog by. "That's just for people who've been athletic all their life," they say. "Exercise is for young people; it would do me more harm than good." "To stay in shape, you've got to work out a couple of hours every day; I don't have time." "I have less energy now than ever before. How could I possibly try doing more?"

These excuses are based on certain prevalent myths

about exercise. Some are entirely untrue; some are half-truths. It wasn't until several decades ago that scientists and physicians began studying the physiology of exercise for people of any age. Virtually all of the initial studies focused on young and middle-aged persons. Very little was known about the promises and perils of exercise for men and women over 50.

Some Myths About Exercise

Fancy: Hard work makes you old before your time.
Fact: Working to exhaustion day after day can wear anyone out. But a regular exercise program actually produces changes in body composition and capacity that run counter to the trends usually seen in aging.

———————————

Fancy: Exercise can lead to a heart attack.
Fact: A sudden burst of intense physical activity after years of sedentary living could put too much strain on your heart. But regular, reasonable exercise develops stronger, healthier heart muscles and seems to ward off heart attacks.

———————————

Fancy: To get into shape and stay there, you have to work out for hours every day.
Fact: Research has shown that older persons need exercise only three to five times a week for a minimum of twenty minutes a session to maintain fitness.

———————————

Fancy: If a little exercise is good, more is better.
Fact: We have found that persons over 50 need to exercise only to 40 to 60 percent of their capacity to derive

maximum benefits. Overexercising is both dangerous and impractical.

•————————————————•

Fancy: Exercise leaves you exhausted and sore.

Fact: Again, a sudden exercise binge, particularly if you do calisthenics that encourage contraction of the muscles, can wear you out and cause aching muscles. The fitness program presented in this book starts at a level well within your capacity and progresses gradually, and the exercises are designed to stretch your muscles and prevent aches and pains. Regular exercise makes you more relaxed, builds your energy reserves, and allows for easier, freer movements.

TURNING BACK THE CLOCK

With support from the federal government's Administration on Aging and the University of Southern California, we set out more than a decade ago to design a safe, effective, scientific fitness program for older people. The site we chose was the Leisure World retirement community in Laguna Hills, California. More than two hundred men and women, aged 56 to 87, participated voluntarily in the research program over five years. Each underwent a thorough physical examination to confirm basic good health, but there were no prerequisites for fitness. Some of the participants had been active all their lives and still played golf and tennis regularly. Others hadn't exercised since their teens, if ever. The fitness program combined a walk-jog routine, calisthenics, and static stretching in hour-long workouts three to five times a week. We tested the volunteers' responses to exercise before, during, and after the sessions.

Six weeks after the program started, we began to see dramatic changes in the participants. Their blood pressure readings dropped. The percentage of body fat decreased. Maximum oxygen capacity increased. Arm strength improved. Electrical activity in the muscles, a sign of nervous tension, diminshed. Most of the volunteers continued to improve, though at a slower rate, for eighteen to forty-two weeks until they reached their peak levels of fitness. Many reported specific and unexpected benefits: A woman plagued by headaches for years no longer needed daily doses of aspirin; her headaches disappeared. A man with chronic lower back pain reported, "I no longer know I have a back." After two months of exercise, a volunteer who'd had continuing problems of irregularity and constipation no longer had to rely on cathartics and laxatives. Troublesome kinks in backs and joints vanished. Some people said they'd never slept better. Several commented that their sex lives were more active than they'd been in years. Even those with mild illnesses improved. A man of 70 who'd had emphysema since age 55 was able to run more than a mile without stopping and to breathe more easily throughout the day.

Regular exercise quite literally turned back the clock for our volunteers. Men and women of 60 and 70 became as fit and energetic as those twenty to thirty years younger. And the ones who improved most were those who had been the least active and the most out of shape. The higher the initial blood pressure measurements, or the percentage of body fat, or the degree of muscular tension, the greater the benefits. The program also proved an important, fundamental point: that it's never too late for fitness. Our oldest volunteer, Walter, was 87 when he signed up. His family, friends, and doctor had one objection: They feared he was too old. We monitored Walter even more carefully than the mere "youngsters" in their sixties and seventies. He not only completed the fitness program but remained active and healthy for years afterward.

Other studies have confirmed our findings: Men and women over 50 are just as capable of exercise and derive just as much benefit from it as the young and middle-aged. For older men and women, exercise has an extra payoff: It slows, stops, and even reverses some of the deterioration associated with aging. Older people who become and remain active may not be reborn, but they certainly are rejuvenated. Exercise lops years off their chronological ages.

How does exercise do this? It increases the strength, endurance, and efficiency of the muscles of the heart, easing its work load. It appears to slow the stiffening of the blood vessels, and some think it may build up networks of small blood vessels through the heart and body to transport oxygen more efficiently. Exercise builds up breathing capacity by expanding the lungs and strengthening the muscles that make them expand and contract. It halts the loss of lean muscle and burns up excess fatty tissue. Joints wear out less quickly if they're exercised regularly, and active older persons have fewer arthritic changes in their hips than sedentary ones. Exercise not only stops mineral loss from bones but also builds up the bone mass. It delays the impact of the aging process on reaction time and movement speed. And it works wonders for mind as well as body: Participants in our program and in others like it reported more energy, less tension, more restful sleep, and fewer feelings of depression and anxiety.

AN ANTI-AGING PILL

Some gerontologists believe that exercise may be the single most effective way to lengthen life. In the largest biological study of human life and death, the American Cancer Society reviewed the habits and histories of more than a million persons over twenty years and found that death rates were significantly higher among those who did not exercise. Mortality rates dropped as exercise increased, and the researchers concluded that exercise warded off heart disease and stroke and helped prolong life. Dr. Alexander Leaf of Harvard Medical School sums up all the evidence for exercise's benefits by saying, "Exercise is the closest thing to an anti-aging pill."

His choice of words is particularly apt. Exercise is as powerful as a drug and should be prescribed and used as carefully as any drug. This book presents a prescription for exercise scientifically designed to meet the ability and needs of people over 50. We do not recommend the high-intensity exertions of younger athletes. Instead, we suggest a combination of different types of exercise—walk-jogging, calisthenics, and static stretching—that require short bursts of low-intensity activity over a relatively long period of time. Through careful, sophisticated tests of the stress that each "dose" of exercise places on the body, we developed self-measuring techniques that you can use to tailor the fitness program to your own level of ability. This exercise prescription is personal, safe, and effective. It requires very little equipment and no special facilities. And to gain these benefits, you need to exercise only three hours a week. By following the instructions step by step, you can prevent the sore muscles you may have developed with other exercises, and you can progress gradually as your capacity for exercise improves.

What can this fitness program mean to you? Think about the years of your future. A man or woman of 50 can look forward to a quarter-century of life. And the longer you live, the longer you can expect to live. Consider some statistics: The life expectancy for the average American male is 69.4 years; for the average female, 77 years. Yet a man who reaches 65 can expect to live another thirteen years. If he makes it to 75, he can look forward to another nine years. A 65-year-old woman has a life expectancy of seventeen years; a 75-year-old woman, twelve years. Sociologists, discussing the "graying" of America, call those under 75 the "young-old" and those over 75 the "old-old." The most senior of citizens are increasing in numbers even more rapidly than the youngsters between 50 and 75. As we head into the twenty-first century, youth may still be served, but the voices that will be heeded most are sure to belong to their elders. And Americans in their fifties, sixties, seventies, eighties, and nineties will have more influence than any of their earlier counterparts in setting the cultural, political, and economic tone of our society.

But quality of life may be far more crucial than quantity. Living well, not simply surviving longer, is our ultimate goal. When the Scripps Foundation for Research in Population Problems asked a sample of Americans over 50 what their highest priority was, the majority said that health, not wealth, mattered most. No other factor was more important to their happiness. Today's men and women over 50 can actually get healthier as they grow older. In our program we've seen men and women in their seventies become more fit and vigorous than they'd ever been before.

What is the state of your own health? Do you worry about high blood pressure and heart troubles? Does a flight of stairs loom before you like Mount Everest? Can you keep trim or are you getting wider as you grow older? Can you move freely or are your joints stiff and sore? Do you sleep well and wake refreshed? Can you relax during the day? Do you have enough energy to carry you into an evening of activity?

We're not saying that this fitness program can or will cure all that ails you. We have not discovered the fabled Fountain of Youth, nor did we ever set out to do so. We know of no way to jog or stretch your way to eternal youth. But this exercise plan has helped many older people look and feel better than before. And even though we can't guarantee that regular exercise will add years to your life, it does hold the rich promise of adding life to your years.

2

Young at Heart

In a long-term study of the health of the people of Framingham, Massachusetts, the U.S. Public Health Service documented the chances of developing heart disease among various groups in the population. Long before any symptoms appeared, epidemiological research could identfiy high-risk groups. Among the highest risk factors are male sex, age over 35, cigarette smoking, high blood pressure, high levels of certain blood fats, and a family history of cardiovascular disorders. Other researchers have added to this list another risk factor: the compulsive, hard-driving, highly anxious personality. The greater the number and severity of any of these risk factors, the greater the person's overall risk.

These threats to the heart can be divided into two main categories: those beyond individual control, such as age, sex, and heredity, and those that can be controlled, avoided, or even eliminated. Among those in the second category are what cardiologists (heart specialists) call "the triple threat": cigarette smoking, high blood pressure, and high cholesterol levels in the blood. If you smoke a pack of cigarettes a day, your risk of having a heart attack is twice that of a nonsmoker. If you smoke, have hypertension, and eat a diet high in fats, your risk is five times greater than normal.

THE HEALTHY HEART

If these risk factors endanger the heart's health, what enhances its well-being and improves its odds of working long and well? Obviously, quitting cigarettes and eating a low-fat diet will help. The next best thing you can do for your heart's sake is to give it what it needs: regular exercise. The heart is a muscle, or, more accurately, a group or "package" of muscles, similar in many ways to the muscles of the arms and legs. And just as exercise strengthens and improves limb muscles, it also enhances the health of the heart muscles. A dramatic case in point is Clarence DeMar, a famous marathon competitor who ran twelve miles every day and competed in marathons at the age of 65. When he died of cancer at age 70, an autopsy showed that this exceptionally strenuous exercise not only had *not* hurt his heart, but had developed and enlarged his heart muscles. His coronary arteries were two to three times normal size.

Since World War II, several large-scale statistical studies have evaluated the relationship between physical activity and cardiovascular disease. One well-known survey compared 31,000 drivers and conductors on London buses. The more sedentary drivers had a significantly higher rate of heart disease than the conductors, who walked around the buses and climbed stairs to the upper level. University of Minnesota researchers did a similar study of railway clerks (in sedentary jobs), switchmen (whose jobs required moderate activity), and section men (who had very active jobs). The section men had a far lower rate of death from heart disease; the clerks were the most likely to die of cardiovascular problems. Other researchers, comparing physically active and inactive workers, have all come to the same conclusion. In the Framingham study, sedentary workers in every age group had almost twice the incidence of heart attacks compared with those who were just moderately active.

The why and how behind these statistics were best explained by classic experiments with dogs whose coronary arteries were surgically narrowed to resemble those of humans with atherosclerosis. Dogs who were exercised had much better blood flow than those kept inactive. The exercise seemed to stimulate the development of new connections between the impaired and the nearly normal blood vessels, so exercised dogs had a better blood supply to all the muscle tissue of the heart. The human heart reacts similarly to supply blood to an area of the heart damaged in a myocardial infarction, a heart attack in which the heart muscle (the myocardium) does not get enough oxygen and other nutrients and begins to die. To enable the damaged heart muscle to heal, the heart relies on new small blood vessels for what is called collateral circulation. These new branches on the arterial trees can develop long before a heart attack—and can prevent a heart attack if the new network takes on enough of the function of the narrowed vessels. Some researchers have observed that exercise can stimulate the development of these life-saving detours in the heart. One study further showed that moderate exercise several times a week is more effective in building up these auxiliary pathways than extremely vigorous exercise done twice as often.

Such research has led some people to think of exercise as a panacea for heart disorders, a fail-safe protection against disease and death. That isn't so. Even marathon runners have suffered heart attacks, and exercise cannot overcome a combination of other risk factors. But as a general rule, exercise helps reduce the risk of harm to the heart. In a recent study of men who graduated from Harvard College between 1916 and 1954, Dr. Ralph Paffenbarger of Stanford University found that the nonexercisers had a 49 percent greater risk of heart attack than their active classmates. He attributed a third of that risk to sedentary life-style alone.

BLOOD PRESSURE: BAROMETER OF HEALTH

Blood pressure is created by contractions of the heart muscle, which pump blood through the miles of blood vessels in the body, and by the resistance of the arterial walls. With each beat of the heart, blood pressure goes up and down within a limited range. It is higher when the heart contracts (a stage known as *systole*) and lower between contractions *(diastole)*. High blood pressure, or hypertension, occurs when the artery walls squeeze down excessively on the blood as it flows. Normal blood pressure in most adults under relaxed conditions should be below 150 systolic (when the heart contracts, putting extra pressure on the blood vessels) and 90 diastolic (when the heart expands and refills with blood, lessening the pressure on the vessels). Blood pressure is measured in millimeters of mercury.

Since the heart functions as a pump, energy demands on it can be increased in one of two ways: by requiring a faster flow rate or by increasing the pressure in the "pipes" or vessels through which the blood circulates. The heart can handle without strain the demand for faster and faster flow. However, greater pressure in the vessels forces it to work harder. In people with chronic hypertension, the heart must work constantly against higher pressure. At the simplest level, such high pressures are hazardous for the same reason that high pressures in an automobile tire are dangerous: the risk of a "blowout" is increased. The human equivalent of a blowout is an aneurysm, a blood-filled bulge in the artery wall that can block or diminish the blood flow to the heart (causing a heart attack) or to the brain (causing a stroke).

Blood pressure is so critical that some cardiologists refer to it as a barometer of health; it can be used to forecast the heart's well-being much as a meteorological barometer aids in predicting weather conditions. The higher the blood pressure readings, the greater the risk. Excessive pressure can lead to serious cardiovascular, kidney, and cerebral problems. It damages the interior walls of the blood vessels, making them more likely to become clogged with deposits of fat, fibrin (a clotting material), cellular debris, and calcium. The arteries themselves lose their flexibility as this sludgelike lining thickens, and blood moves through the narrow channels with increasing difficulty. Changes in the blood itself, triggered by stress, can compound these problems. In one study, anxiety, tension, fear, anger, and hostility all were implicated as factors that increase the blood's tendency to thicken and clot. Stress seems to stimulate biochemical changes that increase oxygen consumption and cause abnormal secretions of the chemicals that control heart rate.

What causes high blood pressure? Sometimes abnormalities of the kidneys are responsible. In his study of Harvard alumni, Paffenbarger identified more common contributing factors: heredity, obesity, and lack of physical activity. What can be done to lower blood pressure? Again, exercise seems to be just what the doctor might order.

In our volunteers, we saw an average of 2.4 percent reduction in systolic and a 4.5 percent drop in diastolic blood pressure measurements. Those with elevated initial readings had the greatest declines. Even relatively normal levels dropped as the exercise program continued. In a six-month fitness program at San Diego State, researchers noted average declines of 12 mm systolic and 13 mm diastolic. When 1,700 men of various ages were surveyed in another test, the more active ones had significantly lower blood pressure readings, regardless of age.

Some Russian scientists suggest that exercise may also have an effect on the walls of the arteries. Their research showed that active men had more elasticity in their blood vessels than did sedentary men.

BLOOD FATS:
GOOD GUYS VERSUS BAD GUYS

Two types of blood fats, or lipids, have been associated with cardiovascular disease. They are cholesterol and triglycerides, both ingredients of essential body chemicals known as lipoproteins. The lipoproteins are divided into four main types: high density, low density, very low density, and chylomicrons. Cardiologists have concentrated on the high-density lipoproteins (HDLs) and the low-density lipoproteins (LDLs). They've dubbed the HDLs the "good guys" because they're found in high levels in people who are not likely to develop heart disease (such as young women and athletes), and the LDLs the "bad guys" because they're found in small quantities in these low-risk people. Some researchers believe that more important than the HDL or LDL levels is the ratio of one to the other; the higher the ratio, the lower the risk of heart trouble.

No one knows precisely how HDL might protect the heart. Researchers believe that LDL is a vehicle for transporting cholesterol into the smooth muscles of the inner artery, where it collects and narrows the passage. HDL may work against this process by resisting the

movement of cholesterol into the arterial wall or by pro-
moting its removal to the liver, where it is broken down
and excreted.

Exercise has a definite effect on how much of these fats
is in the blood. In one recent report in the medical liter-
ature, doctors compared the HDL levels of marathon
runners, joggers, and inactive people. The long-distance
runners had more HDL than the joggers, who had more
than the sedentary men and women. The researchers
concluded that the amount of exercise people get may
have more effect on HDL levels than what they eat. Another study proved that exercise could lower triglyceride
levels by 40 percent—but just for a couple of days. Only
regular exercise can keep down the levels of this harmful
blood fat.

AFTER A HEART ATTACK: COUNTERATTACK

Prevention is always the best medicine, but what can exercise do after damage is done to the heart? There's no
evidence that it can cure or reverse the effects of a heart
attack or of severe atherosclerosis. However, it can relieve the symptoms of heart disease for patients who've
had myocardial infarctions, who suffer from chest pain
(angina), or who've undergone surgery for congenital de-
fects or coronary bypasses. Typically only 40 percent of
patients who survive a heart attack recover sufficiently to
resume their normal work. But 80 percent of those who
undergo rehabilitation either return to their original jobs
or start new positions.

Some researchers say that the best defense after a heart
attack is offense. But rehabilitation must be carefully su-
pervised by a physician and must start slowly, at a level
well below capacity, and progress gradually to longer,
more intense activity. Patients undergoing rehabilitation
cannot expect to reach the same maximum levels of ex-

ertion as a healthy person; instead, their capacity must be based upon their individual symptoms and exercise responses.

Exercise does not have the same training effect on heart disease patients that it does on others. There is no evidence that it either increases collateral circulation or improves the heart's oxygen supply. For patients with chest pain, or angina, its major benefit is building up their tolerance for pain-free activity. Everyday activities that once might have been too much can then be done with relative ease. The reason, doctors believe, is that exercise reduces the heart's demand for oxygen and, therefore, its demands for a greater blood supply. The heart, in a sense, becomes more efficient: it can do more with less.

Other researchers also have good news for recovering heart-surgery patients. They've found that eventually these men and women can achieve the performance levels of normal, sedentary persons. Some cardiac patients come back stronger than ever before as they make exercise part of their routine. A few have gone through special long-distance training programs and competed in marathon races.

SAVING HEARTBEATS

Most hearts beat seventy to seventy-five times each minute. An athlete's heart beats only fifty or fewer times. Every hour the athlete's heart works less hard. Every day it beats 36,000 fewer times; every year it saves 12,960,000 beats; in the course of a lifetime, it subtracts 933,120,000 beats from the average work load on the heart. Saving heartbeats is important for older persons as well as athletes. As we age, pushing our heart rate beyond a safe maximum limit becomes increasingly dangerous. The lower the heart rate, the more we can do within that safety limit.

Take a moderately heavy exercise, one that raises the heartbeat of a well-conditioned 65-year-old man from 60 beats to a comfortable 127 beats per minute. If an unconditioned man of the same age attempted the same activity, he'd probably have to go from his norm of 75 or 80 beats up to his maximum of 160 beats, if not higher—and he'd be exhausted by the all-out effort.

R̥ for a Healthy Heart

The heart and blood vessels respond best to what are known as aerobic exercises. *Aerobic* literally means "with air," and aerobic exercise is the kind in which the amount of oxygen taken into the body is slightly more than or equal to the amount of oxygen used by the body. Sustained, nonstop activity, such as walking or jogging, helps the heart because:

- It lowers the blood pressure. In our fitness program, even relatively normal blood pressure readings declined. The greatest improvements were seen in volunteers with previously high blood pressure measurements.
- It builds up auxiliary networks of small blood vessels to lessen the load on the arteries.
- It raises the levels of high-density lipoproteins (HDLs), which scientists believe are important in slowing or resisting the buildup of cholesterol in the arteries.
- It increases the amount of oxygen consumed per heartbeat, so the heart needs to beat less frequently per minute.
- It helps patients who have had heart attacks return to the same performance levels as healthy, sedentary persons.

Paradoxically, the best way to bring your resting heart rate down is to push it up during regular exercise. By forcing your heart toward its potential capacity, you train it to transport more oxygen with each beat. In designing a fitness program for older people, we relied on measurements of "oxygen pulse," the amount of oxygen consumed per heartbeat, to determine how much exercise was enough to provide desired benefits. This measurement is proportional to maximum oxygen consumption and is closely correlated with the stroke volume, the volume of blood pumped by the heart at each contraction. As we measured our volunteers' oxygen pulse through the weeks of the program, we were able to document that their hearts were beating and pumping like those of 40- to 50-year-olds. Participants increased the amount of oxygen consumed per heartbeat by 29 percent on the average over a forty-two-week training period. The more oxygen taken in per beat, the fewer beats were required.

THE BREATH OF LIFE

Just as exercise expands the heart's ability to transport oxygen, it also improves the lungs' maximum ventilation capacity and the body's aerobic capacity, the most important indication of our ability to perform work. Until recently, exercise physiologists had not looked into what might be done to bolster the muscles of breathing to increase oxygen intake. Research has now shown that respiratory muscles respond to strength and endurance training by increasing breathing capacity 14 to 55 percent. While exercise cannot restore tissue damaged by chronic obstructive lung disease, it does help to relieve symptoms and improve tolerance for activity by increasing muscle strength and endurance.

In our measurements of improvements in breathing capacity, we noticed a definite difference between the sexes. Even though the women's oxygen-pulse readings improved, their maximum breathing capacity showed little change. By contrast, the men improved by an average of 35 percent; one man increased his breathing capacity by a whopping 129 percent. Why this inequality? The likely explanation involves the chest wall. As men age, the chest wall loses elasticity and creates greater resistance against vigorous breathing. Women do not seem to develop this stiffness. Exercise, by improving elasticity, enabled our men volunteers to breathe more deeply. The difference showed up in our measurements of maximum oxygen consumption.

℞ for Better Breathing

The best indication of how much work or activity we can perform is our maximum oxygen consumption, a measurement of how much oxygen we can take in as we breathe. Sustained aerobic exercise builds up our oxygen consumption because:

- It strengthens the respiratory muscles.
- It increases their endurance.
- It relieves the symptoms of chronic obstructive lung disease.
- It improves the elasticity of the chest wall to make deep breathing easier.

The heart and lungs, the basic mechanisms for sustaining our bodies, are designed to be life-givers, not life threats. They are complex and incredibly durable. By their very nature, however, they can and do wear down and malfunction. Disease is inevitable some of the time, but avoidable a great deal of the time. Your heart belongs to you. No drug, no operation, no miracle cure can do as much for it as you can. In the most fundamental sense, nobody but you can break your heart.

3

Fit or Fat?

When Mike turned 65, he was twenty-five pounds overweight. By strict dieting, he shed the extra pounds, but he lost more than weight; he also lost his energy and vitality. He was always exhausted, and his friends, seeing his gaunt, drawn face, worried about his health.

By the time Mike volunteered for our fitness program two years later, he had put the twenty-five extra pounds back on. After six months of exercise and some willpower at the dinner table, Mike slimmed down again. This time he felt better than he ever had, brimming with energy and glowing with good health.

What made the difference? The first time Mike lost *weight*; the second time he lost *fat*. The distinction is important. According to research, a large portion of the weight lost by dieting alone is active tissue, such as muscle and connective tissue, while a smaller fraction is excess fat. When Mike cut calories drastically to lose weight, he lost active tissue needed to sustain his energy.

Exercise had the opposite effect: It increased his lean body mass and decreased his excess fat.

The numbers on your scale don't indicate whether you're fit or fat. Far more significant than your total body weight is the composition of your body tissue. If a man's fatty tissue is greater than 14 to 15 percent of his body mass, or if a woman's is more than 20 to 22 percent, he or she is overweight—or, more precisely, overfat. A small amount of fat is needed for padding the internal organs and as insulation under the skin. Excess fat leads to such diseases as diabetes, gout, high blood pressure, coronary artery disease, and gallbladder problems. There are very few very fat very old persons. The reason is that the fittest, not the fattest, survive.

The delicate balance between fatty tissue and active tissue (muscles, glands, connective tissue, and internal organs) changes as we age. Each decade after age 25 we lose 3 to 5 percent of our active tissue. Unless we also lose 3 to 5 percent of our total weight, we start getting fatter. If you're 60 years old and weigh as much as you did at 20, you're probably 12 to 15 percent overfat. And you're certainly not alone. Weight problems are typical in our society. We are so far advanced industrially that we can produce and store food in abundance, and all with very little physical effort by most of the population. With more food available, we eat more. But fat is not made by food alone.

Think of the human body as a heat-exchange engine that works on the basic principles of energy physics: The caloric balance equals the total calorie intake minus the total calorie expenditure. Some of the calories we ingest are used for basal metabolism; as we age the body requires fewer calories for this basic upkeep. Some calories are excreted as waste products. Some go into "work metabolism," the energy expenditure required for any physical activity. If we take in more calories than are used by these functions, we have a caloric excess. By the laws of physics, energy is transformed rather than destroyed. In this case, each excess of 3,500 calories is changed into a pound of fat. If we want to reverse this process, we have to burn up 3,500 calories to lose a single pound.

LOSING FAT

Transforming food into fat seems all too easy for most of us. Losing fat is far more difficult, and to accomplish this we have only three alternatives: (1) decrease food intake and keep activity constant, (2) increase activity and keep food intake constant, or (3) combine both approaches— diet and exercise.

Many of us become professional dieters. Year after year, we peel off pounds with the current fad diet—only to put the weight back on after reaching our goal and return to the habits that made us fat in the first place. But we can't blame our fat on food. In one study of the causes of obesity, researchers found that only 3.2 percent of obese people became fat because of increased food intake. In 67.5 percent of the cases, inactivity was associated with the onset of obesity.

Physical activity can help reverse the results of inactivity. An hour of vigorous exercise burns up 300 to 600 calories. If you also cut 300 to 500 calories from your daily menu, you can lose weight at the rate of one to two pounds a week. Without exercise, you'd have to eat 500 to 1,000 fewer calories a day to lose the same number of pounds in a week. Exercise is not for everyone who's overfat, however. The severely obese person should exercise *only* under medical supervision to prevent strain on the cardiovascular system and connective tissue. And no one should restrict food intake drastically without consulting a doctor.

How can you know if you need to lose fat? The best way is by finding out what percentage of your total body mass is fatty tissue. Be wary of the insurance tables that provide ideal weights for men and women of various heights. Rarely do these tables take body types or age into account. A six-foot man with a light skeletal frame could be thirty to forty pounds overweight at 200 pounds; a more muscular man with a heavy skeleton could be at his ideal weight. Weight tables sometimes allow slight increases with increasing age. This is misleading and wrong. Unless you've built up more lean muscle mass through exercise, you should weigh less, not more, as you get older.

Our fitness program did not include a diet plan. Nevertheless, our volunteers lost an average of about 1 percent of body weight. More important, they lost 3.6 percent of their body fat, three times more fat than weight. Those who combined exercise with a cutback in calories lost more fat and more pounds.

WINNING THE WAR AGAINST FAT

When you think of fighting fat with exercise, you probably think of hours of hard, sweaty exertion. In our program, participants never worked at more than 60 percent of their capacity, and the exercise sessions lasted for only an hour. Yet the volunteers not only lost fat during these workouts, but they kept losing fat for hours afterward—without moving a muscle or working up a sweat. How? During exercise they would raise their resting metabolism—one of the functions that burns up calories—by 7.5 to 28 percent. The higher rate persists for at least six hours after exercise. In the course of a year, this post-workout boost in caloric consumption could lead to a loss of four to five pounds—over and above the fat lost during exercise.

If exercise speeds up metabolism, doesn't it also stimulate the appetite? Will you eat more as you exercise more, canceling out the benefits of your workouts? Harvard nutritionist Jean Mayer says no. Appetite does not increase in proportion to moderate activity. Your hunger will increase only if you exercise for more than an hour a day, a period longer than we recommend for persons over 50. In laboratory studies, Mayer found that appetite *decreased* in previously sedentary animals when they were exercised for half an hour to an hour each day. Studies also show that when you eat might be as important as what you eat. Rats trained to eat their entire daily ration in one to two hours gained more weight than rats who nibbled at their food whenever they were hungry. Eating just one giant meal increased the rate at which food is converted into fat by twenty-five times.

Some people are discouraged from exercising to lose fat because they think they have to work off 3,500 calories in one marathon effort. The metabolic equation of 3,500 calories per pound does not dictate the rate at which weight can be gained or lost. You're far better off trying to lose fat a little at a time by adding pleasurable activities to your schedule. Just an extra half-hour of walking, for example, can burn off five pounds a year. Try to think in terms of the long haul and develop eating and exercise habits that can keep you in shape for months, years, and decades to come. This perspective can help you get over one of the very common disappointments of the first weeks of dieting: You step on your scale after one, two, or even three weeks of dieting and exercise, and your weight is still the same as when you started. Don't be discouraged. Body tissues often retain water to offset the weight of the tissues being burned off. This water retention can't and won't last forever. Eventually you'll be able to see the progress you're making.

R̶ for Fat Loss

Exercises that help burn up more calories than you take in can help you lose excess fat. Even if you have a very specific bulge of fat as your target, "spot exercising" will not be more effective than overall conditioning activities. The body naturally sheds fat from the areas of greatest excess. Exercise helps you lose fat because:

- It increases the calories your body uses every day. An hour of vigorous activity burns up 300 to 600 calories (the equivalent of a hamburger and a milk shake).
- It burns up excess fatty tissue while building up lean body mass, so you don't lose vital active tissue. It keeps the percentage of body fat at the appropriate level.
- It raises the metabolic rate for more than six hours after exercise so that your body continues to consume more calories *after* as well as during workouts.
- It decreases appetite if you lead a fairly sedentary life.

4

Aches and Pains

As we age, we begin to complain more of pains in our muscles and joints. We seem to stiffen up with age, and such commonplace activities as bending over for the morning paper can make us wince.

Such pain can grip so fiercely that we're sure it begins deep in our bones. But the real cause of stiffness and soreness lies not in joints or bones, according to researchers at the Johns Hopkins Medical School, but in the muscles and connective tissue that move the joints. The frictional resistance generated by the two rubbing surfaces of bones in the joints is negligible, even in joints damaged by arthritis.

Flexibility is the medical term used to describe the range of a joint's motion from full movement in one direction to full movement in the other. The greater the range of movement, the more flexible the joint. If you can bend forward at the hips and touch your toes with your fingertips, you have good flexibility, or range of motion of the hip joints. But can you bend over easily with a minimal expenditure of energy and force? The exertion required to flex a joint is just as important as its range of possible motion.

Different factors limit the flexibility and ease of movement in different joints. In the elbow and knee, the bony structure itself sets a definite limit. In other joints, such as the ankle, hip, and back, the soft tissue—muscle and connective tissue—limit the motion range. The problem of inflexible joints is similar to the difficulty of opening and closing a gate because of a rarely used and rusty hinge that has become balky. If we don't regularly move our muscles and joints through their full ranges of motion, we lose some of their potential. When we try to move a joint after a long period of inactivity, we feel pain, and that discourages further use. The muscle becomes shortened with prolonged disuse and produces spasms and cramps that can be irritating and extremely painful. The immobilization of muscles, as researchers have demonstrated with laboratory animals, brings about biochemical changes in the tissue.

Until they ache, we tend to ignore our muscles and connective tissue, even though they are what quite literally holds the body together. Connective tissue binds muscle to bone by tendons, binds bone to bone by ligaments, and covers and unites muscles with sheaths called fasciae. With age, the tendons, ligaments, and fasciae become less extensible. The tendons, with their densely packed fibers, are the most difficult to stretch. The easiest are the fasciae. But if they aren't stretched to improve joint mobility, the fasciae shorten, placing undue pressure on the nerve pathways in the muscle fasciae. Many aches and pains are the result of nerve impulses traveling along these pressured pathways.

THE SPASM THEORY

Muscle pain can be excruciating, owing to the body's reaction to a cramp or ache. In this reaction, called the splinting reflex, the body automatically immobilizes a sore muscle by making it contract. Thus a sore muscle can set off a vicious cycle of pain. First, an unused muscle becomes sore from exercise or being held in an unusual position. The body then responds with the splinting reflex, shortening the connective tissue around the muscle. This causes more pain, and eventually the whole area is aching. One of the most common sites for this problem is the lower back.

In the physiology laboratory at the University of Southern California, we set out to learn more about this cycle of pain. Using electromyography (EMG) equipment, we measured electrical activity in the muscles. We knew that normal, well-relaxed muscles produce no electrical activity, whereas muscles that are not fully relaxed show considerable activity. In one experiment we measured these electrical signals in the muscles of persons with athletic injuries, first with the muscle immobilized and then after the muscle had been stretched. In almost every case, exercises that stretched or lengthened the muscle diminished electrical activity and relieved pain, either totally or partially. In other tests, we measured electrical signals before, during, and after inducing muscle pain in volunteers; again, stretching quieted the electrical activity and relieved the pain.

These experiments led to the "spasm theory," an explanation of the development and persistence of muscle pain in the absence of any obvious cause, such as traumatic injury. According to this theory, a muscle that is overworked or is used in a strange position (which forces some fibers of the muscle to overwork) becomes fatigued and, as a result, cannot relax fully. (This is a well-known phenomenon in muscle physiology.) The areas within the muscle that aren't fully relaxed cause a local restriction of blood flow because of increased mechanical pressure on the small blood vessels. The relatively inadequate blood flow, called ischemia, causes muscle pain. The pain triggers the typical splinting reflex and contraction of the muscle. This is what induces the pain cycle: The original pain causes ischemic pain, which causes local muscle contraction, which causes more ischemic pain, and so on. Many of the mysterious aches and pains of aging may be the result of this process.

Permanent relief requires a single break in this pain cycle. In order to accomplish that, we have to understand the two basic stretch reflexes in our muscles: *postural* and *inverse myotatic*. The postural reflex we know best is the one that doctors test by striking the knee (or patella) with a rubber-tipped hammer. The blow lengthens (stretches) the muscle in the upper leg, and in reaction to this lengthening, the postural reflex causes the muscle to contract. If the lower leg swings forward, the "patellar stretch reflex" is intact. The postural reflexes are designed to maintain upright position without any conscious effort. If we start falling forward, the muscles in the backs of our legs are stretched; instantly the postural reflexes shorten these muscles to return us to an erect position. Usually these reflexes respond to quick stretches.

The inverse myotatic reflex responds to static, slow stretching and results in relaxation rather than contraction. Instead of counteracting the lengthening of a muscle (as a postural reflex does), an inverse myotatic reflex helps the muscle lengthen and, once it is in position, holds the stretch. Static stretching relies on the inverse myotatic reflexes to relax muscles and avoid postural reflexes that only aggravate pained muscles. Used very gently but with sufficient force, the static stretch can break up the muscle spasm and relieve pain.

AN END TO SORE MUSCLES

Suppose that at a distance you see a short, stooped figure walking with short, slow steps. Most likely you will conclude that the person is old. The hunched posture gives you the clue. Why does aging contort so many bodies in this way? The reason is that many people, throughout their lives, never extend the neck to its full range, and so the muscles shorten. Long hours of reading, sewing, typing, or standing at a workbench take their toll. Eventually deposits of calcium salts in the joints complete the process of immobilization. Once this calcification takes place, nothing can be done to reverse it.

Fortunately, older persons can take action before it's too late. The best action is regular exercise that stretches the muscles and improves flexibility. Once researchers thought that only young people's joints would respond to such exercise. In one experiment at the University of Southern California laboratory, a doctoral student proved them wrong: She studied twenty older men and twenty younger men as they completed a program of finger exercises. Men in both age groups increased the flexibility of their finger joints (a particularly common sore spot in people over 50), and the old improved as much as the young. But a man or woman over 50 shouldn't try to stretch his or her muscles with the quick, jerky movements that younger people use. These quick bounces can set off the pain cycle, and even minor aches have a way of growing into major pains in older people. Our experiments have shown that there is no need to risk such soreness; static, slow stretching is just as effective in relieving stiffness and enhancing flexibility. (Static stretching exercises are outlined in Chapter 9.)

Aging takes a toll on our bones as well as our muscles: They lose minerals, soften, and shrink. The problem is extremely severe in postmenopausal women; an estimated 40 million suffer from the bone deterioration known as osteoporosis. As the bones lose minerals, they become more fragile, and even a slight fall can lead to a serious fracture. Several studies have shown that this loss can be halted and even reversed. One experiment compared two groups of women with a mean age of 82; one group exercised regularly, while the other group remained inactive. The exercisers *gained* 4.2 percent in bone mineral composition; the sedentary women, in the same period of time, *lost* 2.5 percent of their bone mass.

℞ for Aches and Pains

Static stretching exercises are best for the muscles and connective tissue of older persons because:

- They do not cause sore aching muscles (as do the quick, bouncing exercises that rely on jerky muscle contraction).
- They lengthen muscles that have contracted as a result of pain.
- They decrease the electrical activity in the muscles, a sign that the muscle is in spasm or not fully relaxed.
- They relieve the pain caused by muscle spasm.
- They prevent pain from vigorous exercise if they are included at the end of each workout.

We don't have to allow age and inactivity to resculpt our bodies, making us shorter, fatter, and stiffer with each passing decade. Regular exercise can prevent these changes before they even begin. And we shouldn't accept aches and soreness as inevitable consequences of aging. Consider Andy, a 102-year-old man who went to his doctor because of a pain in his left leg.

"Gee, Andy," the physician said, "what do you expect at your age?"

"Well," Andy replied, "my right leg's 102 too, and it doesn't hurt a bit."

5

Fatigue:
Your Energy Crisis

"I feel like the character in the old joke: My get-up-and-go got up and went." Barbara smiles as she speaks, but for her and millions of other older Americans, chronic tiredness is no laughing matter. An hour's shopping wears her out. She yawns through the trips she and her husband had looked forward to for years. "I can't understand it," she says. "I do less than I've ever done during the day, yet I have less energy in the evening."

Barbara blames her fatigue on "tired blood" or other vague side effects of age. But the real culprit isn't her age; it is her new leisurely life-style. Her body has grown so unused to activity that it tires at the slightest effort. The cure for such weariness isn't a pep pill or a multivitamin but healthy, regular doses of activity.

When we asked the volunteers in our fitness program what they considered the greatest personal benefit of exercise, their most frequent answer was greater energy. As they conditioned their bodies, they tired less during and after the workouts. They had more energy for normal daily activities and enough extra energy for new and different interests. How could more effort lead to more energy? The explanation lies in the way the body's own balance of supply and demand responds to an internal energy crisis.

FUEL SUPPLIES

Food is the body's fuel. Different types of foods—proteins, fats, and carbohydrates—play different roles in nourishing the body. Neither proteins nor fats, although essential in the daily diet, are good sources of the type of energy needed for activity. Work and exercise rely on glycogen, a substance produced by the body from complex carbohydrates and stored in the muscles and liver. The supply of glycogen in the muscles determines and limits the duration of activity. Exercise depletes the glycogen in the muscles and leads to fatigue. But when glycogen is depleted by strenuous activity, it is replaced in quantities greater than before, as if the body recognized the need to lay in a larger supply of fuel. In unused muscles, glycogen levels remain the same; in exercised muscles, they more than double. In a sense, glycogen reserves are like a pile of logs for the fireplace. The number of logs determines how long the fire can burn. When you realize that you'll be relying on the fireplace to provide more heat, you make sure you have more logs on the pile.

Even with plenty of logs, you can't start or sustain a fire without oxygen. The body is the same way. It's impossible to continue physical activity for more than a minute or two without oxygen. Oxidation is essential for converting glycogen to the energy we need to wiggle a finger, flex a muscle, or run a marathon. And oxygen must be available where it's needed—at the individual muscles—to allow for intense activity. The combination of increased glycogen and increased oxygen gives us the energy needed to work longer and more intensely.

MORE MIGHT FOR THE MUSCLES

As a muscle becomes fatigued, it produces less force. To accomplish a task—climbing stairs, for example, or shoveling snow—more units of muscle must be called into play to back up the wearied muscles. The tired muscles are both less efficient and less effective. But muscles can reach the point of fatigue without all-out physical exertion. Even when you sit or stand, some muscles are working, and such relatively easy postures can tax some muscles and cause fatigue. The muscles of the lower back, for example, can be fatigued by the effort of keeping erect when you stand still for several hours. As soon as they become fatigued, they call for help from other muscles.

Muscles in poor condition tire most readily. Consider Joe and Sally, both 63 years old and both in good general health. They set off on a bicycle trip. After a mile, Joe has pushed his muscles to exhaustion; he is trying to muster all the reserves of his body to keep going. Sally, with muscles conditioned by regular exercise, is pedaling vigorously a mile down the road; she won't grow weary for several more miles.

Exercise improves the condition of muscles and their ability to work longer without fatigue. In our laboratory studies of muscles at work, we found that the better conditioned a muscle is, the slower its rate of recruitment of other muscles to help sustain physical activity. Better-conditioned muscles can do more with less before they need to call in the reserves.

In our fitness program, we were surprised to see how quickly the volunteers improved their muscular efficiency and endurance. Just a few weeks of regular activity built up their energy reserves. And the ones who improved most were those who started out in the poorest condition. To test and record their progress, we used a stationary bicycle and increased the work load (the effort required to pedal) every two minutes until the participants were working at approximately 85 percent of their maximum heart rate. With continued training, some of the men and women increased their capacity for pedaling longer and harder by 50 percent.

℞ for More Energy

Vigorous exercise, including calisthenics and sustained activities like walking and jogging, builds up energy because:

- It increases the supply of glycogen (the fuel for physical activity) in the muscles, to sustain longer activity.
- It increases the oxygen available at the muscles to allow for more intense activity.
- It conditions a muscle so that it can do more before it becomes fatigued.
- It slows the rate at which fatigued muscles recruit others to accomplish a task.

6

Stress:
The Wear and Tear
of Tension

We often hear of a type of energy that has little to do with muscles and work, an energy without focus or function: "nervous" energy. We recognize it by any number of other names: stress, anxiety, tension, feeling uptight. Older persons have no monopoly on this sense of malaise. Each year Americans of all ages spend more than $300 million on tranquilizers and sedatives to soothe their fraying nerves.

Stress is a twentieth-century phenomenon, the price we pay for living in our high-powered, fast-paced world. In the short term, we may pay the price in headaches, heartburn, sleepless nights, and stiff, aching muscles. In the long run, the price gets higher. Stress has been implicated as a contributing factor in conditions that range from alcoholism to hypertension, from arthritis to impotence. Its effects are cumulative. Whereas episodes of intense stress affect our immediate well-being, decades of life under pressure affect how long and how well we continue to live.

Stress isn't always negative. Some of life's happiest moments—births, weddings, reunions, retirements—are enormously stressful. Stress is a spice of life, a motivating force for growth and adaptation. But our bodies cannot differentiate between positive and negative stresses, between genuine threats and vague anxieties. Dr. Hans Selye, a pioneer of psychosomatic medicine and the first to use the term *stress* in its current context, defined stress as "the nonspecific response of the body to any demand made upon it." Whatever the stressor, the body reacts with what Selye describes as the "general adaptation syndrome."

It begins with alarm. The muscles, particularly in the face and neck, tighten. The stomach feels knotted. The pulse is rapid, the mouth is dry, and the palms are sweaty. Lactate, a substance released during muscle contractions, appears in the blood. Hormones that speed up the heart and constrict the blood vessels are released. Blood pressure rises.

After this initial response, the body returns to normal, but maintaining normalcy under stress requires all the energy of mind and body. If the stress continues long enough, normal functioning cannot be maintained, and the initial alarm responses reappear. Even a small amount of additional stress at this stage can cause a breakdown. In small animals, stress beyond the point of endurance has proven deadly.

This reaction pattern served our ancestors well. In prehistoric times, people confronted by a dangerous animal had only two options: fight or flight. The body's response to this stress mobilized all their internal resources so that they could do either. These responses still come in handy. If you step off a curb into the path of a speeding car, your body reacts instantly: You jump back to safety in a leap farther and faster than one made when you're not under stress.

Yet quite often our Stone Age bodies respond inappropriately to Space Age stresses. Rarely do we require physical mobilization to cope with the dozens of daily stresses of modern life. Many of these are personal. As researchers have shown, the greatest stresses are events such as the death of a spouse, divorce, or any change in job or location. The world around us adds to these stresses. It is too much with us—too noisy, too crowded, too dangerous, too complicated, too frustrating. Think of what's involved in the everyday activity of driving on the freeway. Safety depends on constant alertness, careful observations, rapid-fire decisions, and considerable guesswork about the intentions of other drivers. Simply getting from home to supermarket and back again could cause enough stress to make a caveman opt for the simplicity of fight or flight.

NERVE ACTION: ALL OR NOTHING

Yet, despite constant and chaotic stresses, we cope. And most of the time we cope very well indeed. By why is it that we react calmly to stress one day and respond with rage a few days later? You can see the same differences in a crowd of people when a child sets off a firecracker. Some are mildly irritated. Some cry out in fear. Some yell angrily at the child.

Physiologists explain these day-to-day, person-to-person differences in terms of the all-or-none law. Every nerve cell, or neuron, responds either to maximum capacity or not at all. Like a rifle, a neuron either fires or doesn't. An overstimulated neuron is like a rifle with the safety switch off. Even a slight stimulus can startle it from a quiet to an active state. A sudden sound—like a firecracker—triggers the startle reflex and sets off many nerve cells at once, literally bombarding the nervous system. And so we overreact, screaming rather than speaking, jumping into the air rather than just stepping backward.

The more active the nervous system, the more active it's likely to become. This cycle of reactions is caused by the feedback mechanisms of the sensory receptors in the muscles. These receptors send back to the central nervous system information on what the muscles are doing, essential data for coordinated movements. As the nervous system becomes hyperactive, the receptors in the muscles become more sensitive. They send more and more information to the nervous system. That is why nervous tension is so often perceived as muscle tension and why a tense person moves stiffly. The muscle receptors have been caught up in the snarl of the overstimulated, overworked nervous system.

Minute changes in the electrical activity within the muscles occur with any activity, even those we barely perceive. Electromyographic instruments can gauge the level of nervous tension by measuring the degree of electrical changes in the muscles. The more electrical impulses in the muscles, the higher the tension level is. We used this technique to measure electrical activity in our volunteers before and after they started the fitness program. Our recordings demonstrated that exercise calms overstimulated nerves.

THE TRANQUILIZER EFFECT

The level of electrical activity in the muscles of our volunteers was low to begin with, about half the average for college-age men and women. With regular exercise, it dropped by 10 percent. One participant, a 68-year-old retired manufacturing jeweler, was particularly tense and had suffered severe tension headaches for years. On initial testing, his electrical activity was higher than the average. After five months of exercise, it dropped 37 percent, and his headaches, which had occurred three to four times a week, vanished. As he put it, he no longer "ate aspirin like peanuts." About this time he went on vacation and traveled for ten days without exercising. The headaches returned; as soon as he started exercising again, they disappeared.

In another experiment, we asked for volunteers who considered themselves extremely nervous. Each person tried several different approaches to relaxation: no treatment at all, a tranquilizer, a placebo (an inactive chemical, or sugar pill), fifteen minutes of walking at a heart rate of 100 beats per minute, and fifteen minutes of walking at a heart rate of 120 beats per minute. Neither the single tranquilizer pill nor the placebo was significantly better than no treatment at all. But exercise did reduce electrical muscle activity from 20 to 25 percent for at least an hour and a half after the workout—at both lower and higher heart rates.

Of course, larger doses of tranquilizers can and do work. But their side effects, including problems of perception and reaction, are especially hazardous for men and women over 50, whose reaction times and movements have already been slowed by age. Dose to dose, exercise is more effective and far safer. And you don't have to worry about how it may interact with other medication you may be taking for medical problems.

How does exercise act as a tranquilizer? Scientists don't understand the precise how and why yet. They believe that certain brain chemicals found in relaxed states are released during exercise. In experiments with cats, researchers found that the activity of the muscle receptors was reduced when the temperature of the receptors themselves or of the hypothalamus, a region in the brain, was raised. Vigorous exercise is one way of raising these temperatures—and, perhaps, of slowing the receptors' activity. Some investigators suggest that the tightening of the muscles associated with tension causes chronic overarousal and overactivity of the nervous system. Moving the muscles, they say, may be necessary to keep the muscle receptors' transmissions to the nervous system at a normal level.

Mental health professionals have begun to study the effects of exercise on emotional disturbances. No one is suggesting that we can quite literally run away from our problems, but one psychologist did find that depressed patients improved significantly after ten weeks of jogging. Other studies have shown a correlation between fitness and emotional stability in middle age and have demonstrated improvements in elderly mental patients when exercise was added to their routine.

℞ for Relaxation

Regular exercise helps to relax a tense body and a stressed mind because:

- It decreases the activity of the sensory receptors in the muscle, which send information to the central nervous system. Tension makes these receptors oversensitive so that they bombard the nervous system with electrical impulses.
- It cuts down on the overload on the nervous system by quieting the electrical signals from the muscles.
- It helps to lift depression and improve mood.
- It enhances the ability to sleep restfully.

Doctors and scientists are just beginning to explore the complex relationship between body and mind. Their research has already shown that the mind acts on the body in countless subtle ways. The preliminary studies of exercise's impact on energy reserves and on persons under stress suggest that the links between body and mind may work in both directions—and that activity of the body can affect the states of the mind.

Part
II

YOUR
FITNESS
PRESCRIPTION

7

Exercise Preliminaries

Prescribing a medication is a complex process. Before physicians decide which dose of which drug can best treat a condition, they consider the patient's age, general health, tolerance for certain medications, and any other drugs the patient may be taking. They check the type of drug, the concentration of active ingredients, the ways it can be administered, and the frequency and duration of its use. To be as scientific and precise as possible, they can consult the *Physicians Desk Reference,* a volume of prescribing information, or the *U.S. Pharmacopoeia,* the most authoritative source of data on the preparation and use of drugs.

Prescribing exercise, as either preventive medicine or therapy, has to be just as scientific and precise, even though physiologists are still developing a compendium of data that could compare to the physician's pharmacopoeia. The type, intensity, frequency, and duration of a "dose" of exercise are all critical. One person's healthy, vigorous workout could be hazardous to another. These dangers may be greater in persons over 50 because they're more likely to have undetected, asymptomatic cardiovascular disease, particularly severe atherosclerosis. Aging also alters the way people respond to activity and to medications and slows their reaction and movement times.

THE SCIENCE OF PRESCRIBING EXERCISE

When we designed our fitness program, we knew that we needed a scientific basis for the prescription of exercise. We needed to know how much exercise would be enough to provide definite improvements, how much might be too much, and how to tailor the activities to individual needs and capacities in a scientific way.

We knew that the stress of exercise could be measured easily. In the normal individual, the rise in heart rate during any physical activity is directly proportional to the stress imposed on the heart, lungs, and blood vessels. Using this measure, and correlating such factors as age, physical fitness, and type and rate of exercise, we produced graphs and tables that became the basis for our fitness plan and largely eliminated guesswork. With these data we could design a personalized exercise program to produce just enough of a physical challenge to bring about a beneficial training effect but not enough to be hazardous in any way.

The first step for every participant would have to be a thorough medical examination. This is essential to guarantee the safety of older people—even so-called "healthy normals"—in an endurance-type exercise program. We also realized that different types of exercise elicit very different physiologic responses, so we had to determine which of the various exercises would be best for men and women over 50.

We were particularly concerned about exercises that might increase blood pressure, a definite risk in older people. European scientists had found that exercises that require muscle contractions, which squeeze down the blood vessels within the tissue, create more marked and undesirable pressure elevations. Higher pressures are needed for the blood to get through the area. This localized blood pressure can "reset" the central mechanism for total blood pressure to a new higher level. Isometric exercises, which maintain muscle contractions in a stationary position for a prolonged time, cause the greatest elevations. We found that crawling exercises and cycling both create isometric tension. The activities that require the least cardiac effort and do not push blood pressure levels up are those in which each muscle contraction is followed by a relaxation. In walking and running, for example, there isn't time during the period of contraction for blood pressure to build. These exercises also maximize the rhythmic activity of the large muscles and minimize the high activation of small muscle masses. We determined that a combination of walking and jogging would be easiest, safest, and most beneficial for persons over 50.

Our next question was how much activity would be enough without any danger of becoming too much. To find the answer, we placed electrocardiographic (ECG) electrodes on the chest of each of our volunteers. They were connected to a small FM radio transmitter that was strapped around the waist. The transmitter sent readings of the heart rate to a recorder while each person exercised. With this system we could observe each individual's response to activity and see exactly what response each dose of exercise stimulated. We found that, on the average, working at 40 percent of the heart's capacity was the minimum for improvements. The best target for exercise was 60 percent. The upper limit—never to be exceeded—was 75 percent.

As we monitored our volunteers over time, we could see improvements in their capacity to do more. Activity that at first seemed hard became too easy with time and repeated exercise sessions. These observations helped us plan for gradual progression in the fitness program. At the beginning of the program, the activities are well within capacity. Slowly we increased the work load from an initial level for unconditioned men and women to a second level for those who had built up their strength and endurance.

Once each volunteer reached peak fitness, we found that relatively little exercise was needed to maintain this state. Just three hours a week—a tiny fraction of the average person's 112 waking hours—could keep heart, lungs, and muscles in top shape. Regular static stretching at the end of each workout, we found, prevented sore muscles and improved flexibility.

WRITING YOUR OWN
EXERCISE PRESCRIPTION

Our fitness program has three basic components:

1. Endurance exercises to condition the heart, lungs, and blood vessels and to induce relaxation. These begin with a carefully planned walking and/or jogging regimen, depending on fitness level.
2. Exercises to strengthen the muscles, particularly those important to good posture. These include calisthenics selected for older men and women.
3. Exercises to improve joint mobility and prevent or relieve aches and pains. These consist of a series of static stretching positions that are safe and effective for older persons.

The following chapter teaches you the self-testing techniques that enable you to tailor this program to fit your fitness level and to measure your progress. Personal record charts are given in Appendix 2, for you to make copies of and use to keep track of your progress. But before you start following the step-by-step instructions, we suggest that you review the following general principles. They are the basics behind your exercise prescriptions.

See Your Doctor. Check with your doctor before beginning the program. If you make any significant changes in your level of physical activity—particularly if those changes could make large and sudden demands on your circulatory system—check with the doctor again.

Take It Slow. Start at a low, comfortable level of exertion and progress gradually. The program is designed in two stages to allow for a progressive increase in activity.

Know Your Limit. By using the self-testing methods described in the next chapter, you'll be able to determine your safety limit for exertion. Stay within it. Overexercising is both dangerous and unnecessary. Use other clues—such as sleep problems or fatigue the day after a workout—to check on whether you're overdoing it.

Exercise Regularly. You need to work out a minimum of three times a week and a maximum of five times a week to get the most benefit. Once you're in peak condition, a single workout a week can maintain the muscular benefits. However, cardiovascular fitness requires more frequent activity.

Exercise at a Rate Within Your Capacity. The optimum benefits for older exercisers are produced by exercise at 40 to 60 percent of capacity. At the beginning of the program, you may want to exercise for a longer period (sixty minutes or more) at a lower intensity. Eventually you can derive as much benefit from just twenty minutes of more intense work.

Warm Up Before You Work Out. To protect your muscles, ligaments, and joints, begin every session with exercises that gradually increase blood flow, and thereby increase the temperature of the local tissue and of the body. This gradual start prevents aches, pains, and injuries. Both muscles and connective tissues are most easily injured then they're cold.

Cool Down After a Workout. The transition from vigorous exercise back to the resting state should be gradual. The circulatory system needs to readjust; the reflexes that open up the circulation during vigorous activity don't reverse quickly when exercise stops. If you go abruptly from strenuous effort to complete inactivity, your muscles, which normally pump blood back to the heart, are turned off. The circulation system can't rely on auxiliary help from the muscles to get blood to the heart. With less blood available, the heart beats more weakly, and blood pressure drops. In some people the drop can be so dramatic that the flow of blood to the brain slows, and they pass out. Usually two to three minutes of walking after you jog is enough to slow you down.

Don't Head for the Shower Immediately. A hot shower opens up the circulation, just as vigorous activity does. Delay your postworkout shower until your circulation system has returned to normal—at least five to ten minutes. Even then, make the shower warm, not hot.

Don't Compete in Conditioning. If you exercise with others, each of you is responding to exercise in a different way. Never compete, except with yourself to bolster your improvements. And never overexert yourself. Overdoing stimulates adrenaline, which makes your heart work less efficiently.

Don't Exercise When You're Sick. Exercise challenges your system to reach its full potential. If you have even a slight cold, your system is already facing a different type of challenge. The double challenge can be too much. You won't derive any benefits by exercising when you're ill. In fact, you might slow down your conditioning progress *and* delay your recovery. Don't resume your exercise program until your energy is back to normal. Until then, concentrate on getting better—and that means taking plenty of rest and following the doctor's orders.

8

Self-testing

Exercise is always a do-it-yourself venture. No other person and no machine can do it for you. But the exercise plans that work fine for people in their twenties and thirties may not be safe or beneficial for you. Our fitness program is tailored to suit men and women over 50, but only you can plan and pace the program to meet your individual abilities and needs. The first step in writing an exercise prescription for yourself is learning more about your body and how to assess its state of health.

STEP ONE:
TAKING YOUR PULSE

Your heart rate is the best measure of your response to various kinds of exercise, and you must monitor it frequently to determine how your body is reacting to various doses of exercise. You can find your pulse at any point in the body where an artery can be squeezed against a bony surface. If you've taken a first-aid course, you've learned about these pressure points. The easiest places to measure pulse during or immediately after exercise are at the wrist (the radial pulse) and on the temple (the temporal pulse). (See Figs. 1 and 2, page 62.)

You'll probably be able to find one of these pulses more easily than the other. Once you've learned how to find your pulse easily and *quickly* at the wrist or temple, you can use one of two methods to measure your heart rate. You can use a stopwatch, which you can purchase at little expense at any sporting goods stores, or you can use a wristwatch with a sweep-second hand.

Measuring Heart Rate with a Stopwatch

After you find the artery and establish the rhythm of your heartbeat, start the stopwatch at a chosen pulse beat, which you count as "zero," not "one." You don't count "one" on the first beat because the pulse you feel is only one point in a cycle of events occurring with each heartbeat. If you plan to count the last beat as completing the twentieth cycle, the first cycle must not be counted until its completion—at the second felt beat. The idea is similar to designating a baby as one year old not at birth but after he or she completes a year of life.

After zero, count the successive beats as "one . . . two . . . three" and so on up to twenty. Stop the watch exactly at the twentieth beat. Remember or record this time and turn to Table A in Appendix 1, page 125. You can easily find your heart rate in beats per minute. For example, if your time for twenty beats was 15.4 seconds, the heart rate was seventy-eight beats per minute.

The reason for counting only twenty beats is that the heartbeat returns to its resting rate very rapidly. We are using this measurement to estimate what the heart rate was *during* exercise, so the closer in time to the actual exercise, the smaller the error.

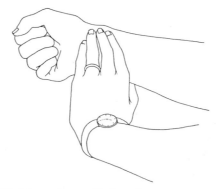

Figure 1. Taking the radial pulse
First locate the large bone on the forearm on the thumb side. This is the radius. Moving inward toward the center of the wrist, you will find a pronounced tendon. Gently place the first three fingers in the hollow between the radius and the tendon; your fingers now are resting on the radial artery. Too much pressure will cut off the flow completely; too little and you won't be able to feel the pulse. Experiment until you find the appropriate pressure to sense the pulse clearly and distinctly. Your hand and wrist should be loose and relaxed.

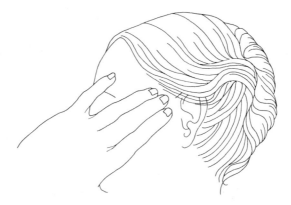

Figure 2. Taking the temporal pulse
Using the left hand for the left artery and the right hand for the right artery, place the first three fingers in the temple—the wide, shallow groove just in front of and slightly above the ear. You should be able to feel a pulse very clearly there.

Measuring Heart Rate with a Wristwatch

After finding the artery and establishing the rhythm of your heart, start the count with "one" on the first beat after the sweep-second hand passes any major mark on the dial, and end the count on the last beat you feel in a ten-second period. You can either multiply by six to get your per-minute heart rate, or you can refer to Table B in Appendix 1, page 127, where the arithmetic has been worked out for you.

Practice often. Once you can get accurate, repeatable resting heart rates quickly and easily, try measuring after exertion. Climb a moderate flight of stairs and have someone time you to see how long it takes you to find the artery and begin the count after you reach the top of the stairs. When you're able to find the artery and begin the count in five seconds or less, you're ready for step two.

We cannot overemphasize the importance of learning how to measure your heart rate accurately. Once you've mastered the technique, you can use it after any activity—mowing the lawn, shoveling snow, or working out—to evaluate the stress on your cardiovascular system. And this reading can tell you something about the *total* stress you're under. For example, if you test your heart rate while gardening on a summer day, you can evaluate the effect on your body of both the exercise and the heat. You've also learned part of the language of medicine, so you'll be able to communicate better with your doctor. Rather than ask your doctor whether it's safe to mow the lawn on a hot day, you can ask whether it's safe for your heart rate to go up to 165. A more specific question gets a more precise answer.

STEP TWO:
MEDICAL APPROVAL

If you haven't checked with your doctor yet, make an appointment now. If you have been getting annual or semiannual checkups and have had one recently, your physician may have enough information to advise you about your capacity for the fitness program over the phone. If not, you should schedule a thorough examination, including such tests of heart function as a resting electrocardiogram and an exercise stress test.

You may want to take this book with you so that the doctor can see the scientific basis for the fitness prescription and the levels of activity for participants. At Level One (Chapter 9), your heart rate won't be pushed beyond 120 beats per minute. In Level Two (Chapter 10), the heart rate limit is 140 for 50- and 60-year-olds and 130 for those over 70. Only your physician can and should decide whether this much exertion is safe for you.

Once your doctor grants medical approval, ask him or her to check on your accuracy in measuring your heart rate. Take your heart rate as you've practiced, and have the doctor take your pulse simultaneously. If three consecutive checks of your resting heart rate show no error greater than three beats per minute, you're doing an adequate job. You might also ask your doctor to check your pulse-taking at a higher heart rate, such as that induced by stepping up from the floor to a low stool and then down again. Under these conditions, your count should be within four beats per minute of your doctor's.

STEP THREE:
ASSESSING YOUR PROGRESS—
THE PROGRESSIVE PULSE RATE TEST

The progressive pulse rate (PPR) test is the basic means of self-assessment. It begins with a very light, slow work load that will not stress the normal older person too severely and should not result in sore muscles. It's done at home and requires no expensive or sophisticated equipment. But you will need some basics: a sturdy kitchen stool (ten to twelve inches high, with a nonslip surface on top and bottom, available in department and hardware stores at a reasonable cost), a stopwatch or a wristwatch with a sweep-second hand, and a cadence counter (either a metronome or a simple pendulum that you can set up— see Fig. 4, page 69).

The entire test consists in stepping on and off the stool in a four-step cycle. Count "one" as you place your left foot on the stool. Count "two" as you lift your entire weight onto the stool by placing your right foot alongside the left. Count "three" as you step down to the floor with your left foot. Count "four" as you bring the right foot back down. To familiarize yourself with the test, practice the four-step cycle slowly. Be sure you are fully extending the knee and hip joints as you stand atop the stool. The test is designed to relate your heart rate to a standard stress, which is measured as the height to which you are raising your body weight. If you don't straighten up, your weight hasn't been raised to the full height of the step and your results won't be accurate. The only other components of the test are timing each step in a specific cadence (by using a metronome or pendulum) and taking your pulse between stool-stepping cycles.

The test consists of four bouts of stool stepping. In the first minute you do twelve four-step cycles (48 steps). In the second minute you do eighteen four-step cycles (72 steps). In the third minute you do twenty-four four-step cycles (96 steps). In the fourth minute you do thirty four-step cycles (120 steps). There's a rest period between each of these bouts.

Set aside one day just for assembling the equipment and practicing the test. Don't rush. If you are setting up a metronome, read all the instructions carefully until you understand them completely. If you are making a pendulum, follow the instructions in Figure 4. Once you're ready, practice the complete test. It's not very compli-

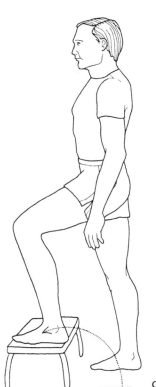

count one   count two

Figure 3. Stool stepping

cated. The key is putting all the factors together and following the procedures in sequence. Since the pendulum swings too quickly for the 48-step series, if you do not have a metronome, you should practice doing a four-step cycle in five seconds, using your watch, until you can keep that pace automatically.

On the day after your setup and practice day, schedule the test for at least one hour after a light meal. To make the test a valid measurement, don't drink coffee, tea, or any other stimulant beforehand and don't smoke or exercise vigorously for several hours before you start. Room

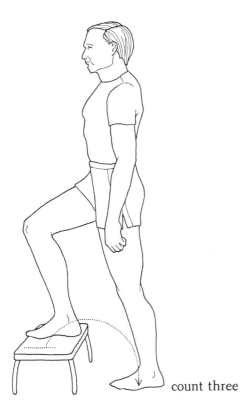
count three

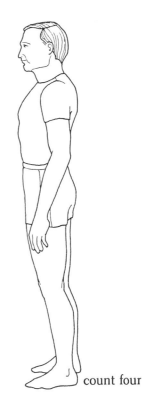
count four

temperature should be between seventy and eighty degrees Fahrenheit. Don't wear binding clothing. Remember to step to the rhythm of the metronome or pendulum; the stress on your system depends on how many times you lift your weight *in one minute*. Chart 1, for recording your progressive pulse rate, can be found in Appendix 2, page 131. Have a copy of the chart and a pencil handy to record the starting point in your fitness program. Set the stool about three feet in front of a comfortable chair. Set up the metronome or pendulum. Hold your stopwatch in your left hand.

The First Minute Bout:
Twelve Complete Four-Step Cycles

1. Seat yourself comfortably and count your resting pulse for thirty seconds.
2. Remain seated for another thirty seconds. Count your resting pulse again.
3. If your pulse is stable (plus or minus two beats per minute in the two pulse counts), multiply the thirty-second count by two to get the minute rate. Circle the minute rate on your chart. If your pulse is not stable, count the sitting pulse again. Continue doing so until two successive counts are the same. If your pulse is still fluctuating after five counts, use the average of the five counts for your resting value.
4. If you are using a metronome, set it to 48 beats per minute. The metronome will click once for each step of twelve four-step cycles in the first minute bout. If you don't have a metronome, use your watch— *not* the pendulum—for the twelve-cycle bout. You will be doing each four-step cycle in five seconds, as indicated by the second hand on your watch.
5. Holding your watch in your left hand, step up with the left foot onto the top of the stool. Take this first step as you start your stopwatch or as the second hand sweeps by the 0 or 30 mark of a wristwatch. Count "one" aloud as you place your left foot on the stool. Count "two" as you place your right foot alongside the left and lift your entire body weight onto the stool. Count "three" as you bring your right foot back to the floor. Count "four" as you bring your left foot down as well. Do twelve complete four-step cycles in one minute.

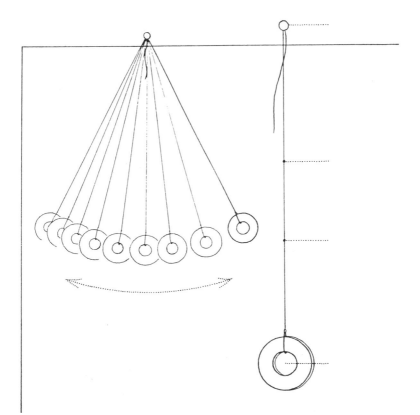

Figure 4. Making your own pendulum

To make a pendulum, simply tie a heavy washer at the end of
a piece of string. Carefully measure from the center of the
washer and mark the string at 9¾ inches, 15 inches, and 27
inches. Tack the string at one of these marks to the top of a
doorframe and set it in motion; if you have measured accurately, your pendulum will swing to its extremes 72 times per
minute when hung from the 27-inch mark, 96 times per minute
when hung from the 15-inch mark, and 120 times per minute
when hung from the 9¾-inch mark. Test your pendulum with
your sweep-second hand or stopwatch. If it is off by more than
a second, try measuring again.

6. As you complete the twelfth four-step cycle at the end of one minute, seat yourself comfortably in the chair and immediately feel for your pulse.
7. Ten seconds after you stop the stool-stepping, start a *two-minute pulse count*.
8. Record the total count for the two-minute period, *not the count per minute*. In the first column of your copy of Chart 1, circle the number that is closest to your two-minute count.
9. Take repeated thirty-second pulse counts until your resting heart rate returns to within ten beats of your original resting rate.

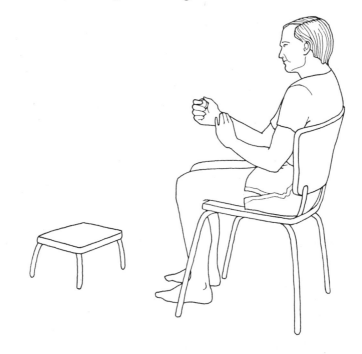

Figure 5. Sit down and count your pulse after completing each stool-stepping cycle.

The Second Minute Bout:
Eighteen Complete Four-Step Cycles

1. Set the metronome to 72 beats per minute. If you're using a pendulum, place the thumbtack through the 27-inch mark (27 inches from center of washer hole to thumbtack) and tack it where it can swing a foot in either direction. Start the metronome or the pendulum swing. Step and count once for each click of the metronome or each time the pendulum swings to each side.
2. Proceed with steps 5 through 9, as in the first minute bout. The only difference is the cadence and number of four-step cycles.

The Third Minute Bout:
Twenty-four Complete Four-Step Cycles

1. Set the metronome to 96 beats per minute. If you're using a pendulum, shorten it so there are 15 inches between the thumbtack and washer center. Start the metronome or the pendulum. Step and count one for each metronome click or each time the pendulum swings to each side.
2. Proceed with steps 5 through 9, as in the first minute bout. Again, the only difference is the cadence and number of four-step cycles.

The Fourth Minute Bout:
Thirty Complete Four-Step Cycles

1. Set the metronome to 120 beats per minute, or shorten the pendulum to the 9¾-inch mark.
2. Proceed as before.

For your first indication of your present fitness, look at your markings on Chart 1. If your score drops by two or more fitness categories as you move to the next higher bout, have someone verify your pulse counts on another day. If your count is confirmed, your exercise results may be abnormal, and you should check with your doctor before continuing the fitness program. The chart in Figure 6 shows a typical, normal response; the one in Figure 7 shows an atypical—but not necessarily abnormal—response in which the heart rate recovery is markedly poorer at higher work loads.

STEP FOUR:
RECORD KEEPING

Using the personal record charts in Appendix 2, you can map your progress in the fitness program. The chart you have just completed marks the starting point. You will retest yourself at six, twelve, and twenty-four weeks after beginning the program and at six-month intervals thereafter. There are also charts for recording your progress in the walking program and in the jog-walk program.

Your personal records are the best and most important indication of whether this exercise prescription is benefiting you. After a year, daily record keeping becomes less important. Unless your doctor asks you to keep up daily records so that he or she can review them during your regular examinations, you can eliminate day-by-day assessments. However, do continue to monitor your progress by the progressive pulse rate test at least every six months. Keep these results to show to your doctor at each routine checkup.

Chart 1. Progressive Pulse Rate Test: Before Conditioning

	Total 2-Minute Pulse Count			
Classification	after 12 4-step cycles per min.	after 18 4-step cycles per min.	after 21 4-step cycles per min.	after 30 4-step cycles per min.
Excellent	102	110	114	125
	106	114	118	130
	110	118	122	135
	114	122	126	140
	118	126	130	145
Above average	122	130	134	150
	126	134	138	155
	130	138	142	160
	134	142	146	165
	138	146	150	170
Average	142	150	154	175
	146	154	158	180
	150	158	162	185
	154	162	166	190
	158	166	170	195
Below average	162	170	174	200
	166	174	178	205
	170	178	182	210
	174	182	186	215
	178	186	190	220
Poor	182	190	194	225
	186	194	198	230
	190	198	202	235
	194	202	206	240
	198	206	210	245

Handwritten annotations circled across the Average row: 148, 151, 161, 174

* Data compiled by Dr. H. A. deVries, K. S. Ambe, and G. M. Adams.

Figure 6. A normal score on the progressive pulse rate test

Chart 1. Progressive Pulse Rate Test: Before Conditioning

	Total 2-Minute Pulse Count			
Classification	after 12 4-step cycles per min.	after 18 4-step cycles per min.	after 21 4-step cycles per min.	after 30 4-step cycles per min.
	102	110	114	125
	106	114	118	130
Excellent	110	118	122	135
	114	122	126	140
	118	126	130	145
	122	130	134	150
	126	134	138	155
Above average	130	138	142	160
	134	142	146	165
	138	146	150	170
	142	150	154	175
	146	154	158	180
Average	150	158 *(161)*	162	185
	154 *(157)*	162	166	190
	158	166	170	195
	162	170	174	200
	166	174	178	205
Below average	170	178	182 *(183)*	210
	174	182	186	215
	178	186	190	220
	182	190	194	225 *(226)*
	186	194	198	230
Poor	190	198	202	235
	194	202	206	240
	198	206	210	245

* Data compiled by Dr. H. A. deVries, K. S. Ambe, and G. M. Adams.

Figure 7. An atypical score on the progressive pulse rate test

STEP FIVE:
GETTING STARTED

Before you plunge into the program, you may have a few questions. Here are the ones we've heard asked more frequently, along with our recommendations.

What's the Best Time to Exercise? Rule out midday because of the heat of the summer months. Mornings and late afternoons are both fine from a physiological viewpoint. However, in practical terms, exercising first thing in the morning is often best. Eat a light breakfast early enough so you'll have time to do your exercise between breakfast and the day's activity.

How Often Should I Exercise? In our program, volunteers exercised three times a week. It may be possible to increase the rate of improvement slightly by upping this to four or five times a week. We recommend a minimum of three and a maximum of five workouts each week. You won't benefit by doing more. Your body needs recharging, much as a battery does.

Where Should I Work Out? Your bedroom is a good site for the calisthenics and stretching exercises. For the progressive walking and the jog-walk, choose the most pleasant surroundings that are available and convenient: a park, beach, recreational area, running track, or schoolyard. Open roads or city streets are equally serviceable but less aesthetically pleasing.

Can I Exercise Year-Round? The progressive walking program can be continued in all but the most inclement weather if you wear appropriate clothing. You'll find your workout particularly invigorating in moderately cold weather or light rain or snow.

What Should I Wear? Your clothing should be loose enough to allow free movement in comfort. For the calisthenics and stretching exercises in your home, loose-fitting casual clothing or undergarments are adequate. For the progressive walking and jog-walk programs, you'll need two layers of clothing so you can peel off the outer layer as you begin to warm up and sweat, and put it back on when you're cooling down. *Sweat* is not a dirty word in this program: you have to sweat if the exercises are to be beneficial.

As basic attire you can wear — in order of preference — a warm-up suit, a sweat suit, or light, loose-fitting casual or work clothes. In summer, you can wear a blouse or T-shirt and walking shorts under the basic attire. In winter, you should add a jacket, coat, or sweater, depending on the weather. Shoes are very important. For the progressive walking, wear sturdy walking shoes with flat heels and sturdy but flexible rubber soles. For the jog-walk, wear good-quality running shoes. Proper fit will prevent blisters.

STEP SIX:
MEASURING THE COURSE

In progressive walking and in the jog-walk program, distance is one way to extend your activity as your condition improves. For this reason, you need to traverse a measured distance. If possible, drive the course and measure the distance with your automobile odometer. If you'll be using a running track, such courses usually are a quarter-mile per lap (for a complete circuit), but check with someone who knows its exact length. If you plan to use a footpath or another course that's difficult to measure by auto odometer, use the following method to determine its length:

1. Measure off a half-mile stretch on a road with an adjacent sidewalk.
2. Walk this half-mile and count the number of paces. (One pace is two steps. Count by the number of times your left foot strikes the ground.)
3. Divide the results by two to get the number of paces per quarter-mile.
4. Use this pace count to mark off a quarter-mile on your course.

STEP SEVEN: STARTING AT THE RIGHT LEVEL

The fitness program has two levels of activity. To find out which one you should start at, look at the progressive pulse rate scores you have recorded on Chart 1, and compare them with the average scores shown on page 73. If you were above average on all four stepping rates, you're ready for Level Two exercises, outlined in Chapter 10. However, read Chapter 9 first because the calisthenics and stretching exercises for both levels are described there. Once you review and learn them, you can move on to Chapter 10.

If you scored in the average or below-average category, start at Level One. The higher you placed on the pulse test, the faster you'll progress in the program. Go slowly at the rate dictated by your heart's response to continued regular exercise.

9

Exercises: Level One

Every workout, at Level One or Level Two, will consist of three parts done in the following order:

1. Progressive walking for Level One; jog-walk for Level Two
2. Calisthenics
3. Static stretching

The order of these activities is critical: The progressive walking or jog-walk provides an almost ideal gradual warm-up before the calisthenics. The calisthenics must be followed by static stretching to prevent muscle soreness, which can otherwise be a major drawback for unconditioned older people.

PROGRESSIVE WALKING

On the first day, take a leisurely walk for half a mile on your measured course, then turn around and walk back to your starting point. If you are in very poor condition, you can shorten even this light load. You should complete the mile walk in twenty minutes. To develop a "pace sense," try coordinating your steps to time and distance requirements. Mark the quarter-mile points as you repeat the exercise on subsequent days. This way you'll be able to note whether you're walking at your planned pace (initially, five minutes per quarter-mile). Check your heart rate at the halfway point. Throughout Level One, you will observe a limit of 120 heart beats per minute. This postexercise rate means that during exercise your heart rate remains below 130. Whenever you find that your heart rate is about 120, slow down the rate of activity.

Record your heart rate on your copy of Chart 2, page 136; for your convenience, you may want to carry this chart on a small clipboard. Table 1 (page 128) outlines your progressive walking goals. The distances and times are approximations. Adjust these as needed according to your heart rate. As the sequence of numbers in the table shows, you'll increase your distance on each of the first nine days. On the first day, you walk a mile in twenty minutes; on the second, you walk 1¼ miles in twenty-five minutes. But if you can't complete the distance on the first day, or if your heart rate goes above your limit of 120 beats per minute, continue working toward the first day's one-mile objective until you reach it without strain. This applies to every day's distance and time goals. Don't attempt to raise your objectives until you have achieved every previous goal.

Increasing the distance makes only very small increases in the demand on your heart. Increasing the intensity (the rate or speed of walking) requires a relatively large acceleration of heart function. The shift from increasing distances to increasing intensity does not occur until the tenth day of the program. At that point you should be capable of walking three miles at the rate of twenty minutes a mile. On day 10 you pick up the pace and walk at the rate of sixteen minutes a mile.

The progressive walking should be fun. Pay attention to your heart rate and your distance goal, but enjoy the scenery as you stride. Whistle, hum, or sing. Swing out with an easy gait, head and chest high, arms relaxed and loose.

If you must walk on a hilly course, keep in mind that walking up even a small grade can multiply the intensity of the required effort. Don't try to adhere to the standard schedule. Let your heart rate be your guide: When walking uphill, take your heart rate at thirty-second intervals. Rest for thirty seconds whenever it reaches 120 beats per minute.

Since walking downhill is less demanding (unless the hill is so steep that your muscles have to work as brakes for your body), try going down first and saving the uphill climb for the end of your walk. If the hill is at all steep, set a comfortable distance of one-half to one mile, depending on the grade. Rather than modify this distance as you progress, decrease the number of rest periods on the uphill climb. When you can make the climb without having to stop to bring your heart rate down to 120, you should be fit enough to increase your walking rate. You may want to increase your uphill distance as it becomes easier for you to walk it at your most rapid pace. "Mountain climbers" can make just as much progress as "flatlanders"—but they do need to use more caution and good sense.

Progressive walking offers a variety of benefits. It builds up the strength and endurance of the heart, lungs, and blood vessels, it has a tranquilizing effect on the nerves, and it burns up calories.

CALISTHENICS

As soon as you complete your walking, begin the calisthenics. Again, your heart rate will determine the rate at which you increase your work load. You will do four different exercises: the bender, the easy push-up, the slow-motion flutter kick, and the easy sit-up. As soon as you finish the easy sit-up, take your heart rate. It should not exceed 120 beats per minute.

If your heart rate is below 120, you can increase the number of times you repeat each exercise at your next workout. But don't increase the number of repetitions to the point of strain or undue fatigue. There is no need to perform these exercises for more than two minutes each. You will improve your fitness by gradually doing more repetitions in the two-minute period.

Do the calisthenics slowly, avoiding any jerky movement. Don't try to force the body further than it will go easily. Don't strain your muscles. (One way to avoid straining movements is to breathe normally throughout. If you find that you need to hold your breath, particularly during the push-ups, you're working too hard. Holding the breath and straining can cause marked and undesirable increases in blood pressure.)

Do the calisthenics indoors. You won't need much room—just enough unobstructed floor space so that you can lie down with your arms outstretched either above your head or to the sides. If the floor is carpeted, you'll need nothing more than a bath towel to put on the carpet for cleanliness. If the floor is bare, either a straw beach mat or a very heavy beach towel should give you a little cushioning (too much is undesirable).

Before you begin, read the instructions carefully and study the illustrations to make sure you understand the movements. Table 2 tells the number of repetitions to start with. Remember to take your heart rate after the fourth exercise.

Exercise 1:
The Bender

The bender is a four-count exercise. Start with feet shoulder-width apart and hands on hips.

Count one: Bend forward gently but firmly and attempt to touch the floor between your feet with your fingers. More slowly. Don't force your hands to the floor.

Count two: Return slowly to the starting position.

Count three: Stretch your arms overhead and bend backward as far as you can *easily* arch your back.

Count four: Return to starting position.

Benefits: As you bend down, the bender stretches the muscles and connective tissue of the upper back, lower back, and hamstring muscles. On count three, the muscles and connective tissue of the abdomen are stretched.

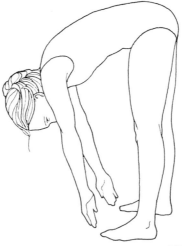

count one

Figure 8. The bender

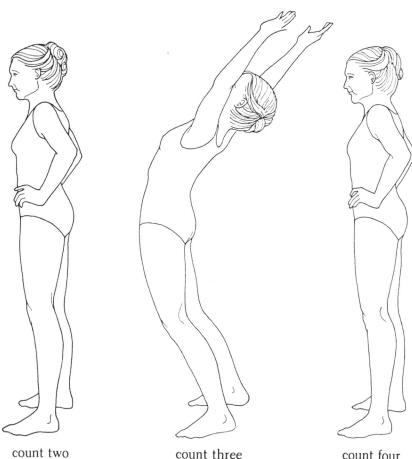

count two   count three   count four

Figure 8. The bender (*Continued*)

Exercise 2:
The Easy Push-up

The easy push-up is a two-count exercise. The easiest way to count during it is: "one-down, two-down. . . ." Start by lying on your belly with your palms flat on the floor alongside your shoulders.

Count one: Straighten the arms, lifting the upper body but leaving the knees and lower legs on the floor. The body should be straight from head to knees.

Count two: Lower the body gently back to the floor.

Keep your breath flowing throughout the exercise. Inhale on the upward movement and exhale on the downward movement.

Benefits: The easy push-up strengthens the muscles of the arms, chest, shoulders, and back—muscles that very few of us use nowadays. At Level One, you must avoid overstraining; take it easy on yourself and your heart by doing only the modified push-up illustrated above during Level One. Women will continue doing the modified form in Level Two.

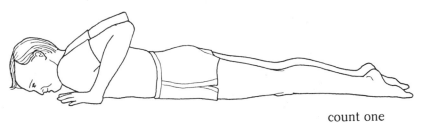

count one

count two

Figure 9. The easy push-up

Exercise 3:
The Slow-motion Flutter Kick

The slow-motion flutter kick is a four-count exercise. Start flat on your belly, with your hands (palms up) under your thighs.

Count one: Lift your head and left leg simultaneously as far as you *easily* can. Keep the leg as straight as possible.

Count two: Return to starting position.

Count three: Repeat with right leg.

Count four: Return to starting position.

Benefits: The slow-motion flutter kick improves the function of the very important muscles of the buttocks and lower back, as well as the hip extensor muscles, which are critical in preventing back problems. This exercise is a sound, safe way to prevent and/or relieve low back pain. It maintains good muscle tone and balances muscular strength appropriately between the front and the back of the body. By enhancing your muscle tone, strength, and endurance, it will also improve your posture and gait.

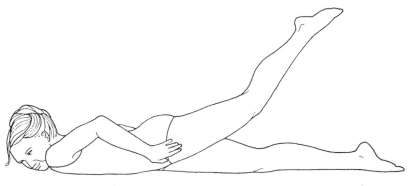

count one

Figure 10. The slow-motion flutter kick

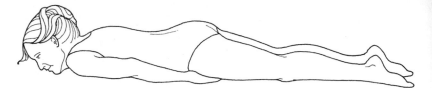

count two

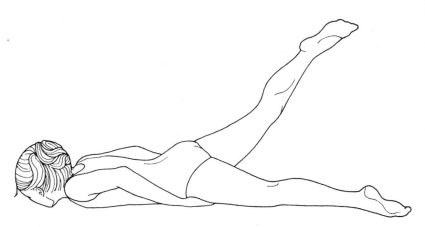

count three

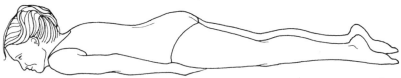
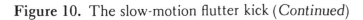

count four

Figure 10. The slow-motion flutter kick (*Continued*)

Exercise 4:
The Easy Sit-up

The easy sit-up is a two-count exercise. Start flat on your back, with your hands (palms down) under the small of your back.

Count one: Lift your head, shoulders, and upper back (as far as your hands) off the floor by tightening the abdominal muscles.

Count two: Return to starting position. (The starting cadence probably will seem slow.)

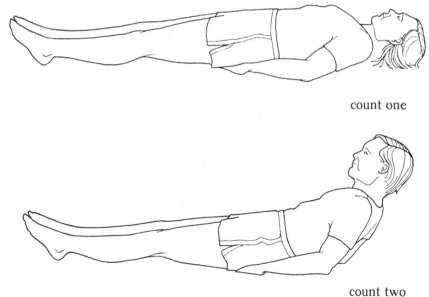

count one

count two

Figure 11. The easy sit-up

Be sure to take your heart rate immediately after this exercise.

Benefits: The easy sit-up improves muscle tone in the abdominal wall, which is important to good posture and may help relieve low back pain of muscular origin. Don't expect this exercise to remove a pot belly, however. Only dietary restriction combined with vigorous activity to burn off calories will do that.

STATIC STRETCHING

Your day's workout ends with a series of nine static stretching exercises designed to cover all the muscles and joints you could possibly have used in the first and second phases of your exercise session. The static stretches bring about their effects through the same basic neurophysiological principles as do the asanas (positions) of yoga; some actually are classic yogic positions. The aims of all are to prevent sore muscles and relieve chronic aches and pains, to improve joint mobility through the safest possible sort of stretching, and to aid in producing a high level of relaxation after a bout of exercise.

Each exercise is illustrated and described in several different levels of increasing difficulty. You are not expected to achieve the most advanced level on the first day, or even in the first weeks or months. Continue doing one intermediate step each day until you can move comfortably on to the next. Remember that the most advanced levels represent your ultimate goal. Work toward that goal in small, easy steps. You might not observe steady progress from day to day, but over a longer period you'll see improvement. How long? That depends on you. If years of inactivity have stiffened your body, it could take a year or longer. If you're overweight, the extra pounds of fat will get in your way and slow your progress.

If you have or have had serious orthopedic problems, discuss the calisthenics and stretching exercises with your physician, who may prefer that you not perform a specific exercise, even though the entire program has been designed for safe use by men and women over 50.

Unlike the other parts of the exercise program, the static stretching exercises can be done to good advantage more than five times a week—even as often as three times a day if time permits. The static stretching drains very little of your energy reserves. You will be working toward the day when you can hold the final position of each exercise for one minute. The more frequently you exercise, the more rapidly you'll progress, although three times a week is sufficient for gradual improvement. If you do the static stretching exercises several times a day, you'll notice that your flexibility improves as the day goes on. This is normal and probably is a result of the progressive loosening up of muscles and connective tissues through use during the day and a tightening up through disuse during the night.

Static stretching must be performed easily and gently, without jerking, bouncing, or sudden movements. Do not hold your breath at any time. When the exercises are performed easily and in the proper manner, they provide an ideal cooling down from the more vigorous parts of the fitness program. They'll leave you invigorated but relaxed.

Exercise 1:
The Upper Trunk Stretcher (Front)

1. Lie flat on your belly, legs straight, toes pointed, forehead on the floor, hands placed down under the shoulders.
2. Starting with your head and neck, arch upward and backward, inhaling as you go upward.

3. Arch the back gradually from the head and neck down as far as the hips.
4. Try to curve your back as much as possible while keeping the hips and legs flat on the floor.
5. Straighten the arms until they're locked.
6. Hold this position for ten to fifteen seconds the first day. Over several weeks or months, increase to one minute. Let yourself down very slowly and easily.

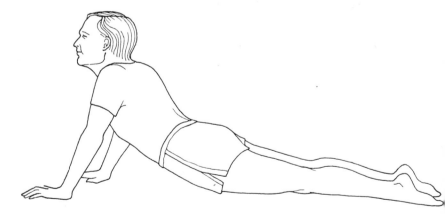

intermediate position

final position

Figure 12. The upper trunk stretcher (front)

Intermediate Steps: To attain this position more easily, three modifications are possible:

    a. Place your hands several inches in front of your shoulders when you start.
    b. Leave the legs slightly apart.
    c. Stop short of full elbow extension in arching the back.

Benefits: This position stretches all the muscles of the upper and front part of the trunk, including the abdominal and trunk muscles. It also strengthens the muscles of the back that extend the spine, improving posture and preventing low back pain of muscular origin.

Exercise 2:
The Lower Trunk Stretcher (Front)

For most men and some women, the lower trunk stretcher position will be difficult to attain. With constant practice, you should reach at least the second intermediate step, although it may require several months of diligent effort. The payoff in better spinal mobility and freedom from pain should make it worthwhile.

Because this position is difficult, everyone should go through the intermediate steps.

Intermediate Step 1: You'll need a belt or small bath towel and two sofa cushions totaling about six inches in thickness.

    1. Kneel on the middle of the two cushions.
    2. Place the belt or towel around your lower legs.
    3. Lie on your abdomen with your knees raised by the cushions, and reach back to grasp the belt or towel with both hands (first one hand and then the other).

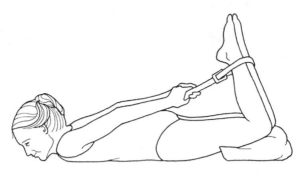

intermediate step 1, with belt and cushions

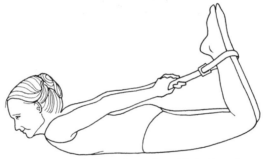

intermediate step 2, with belt only

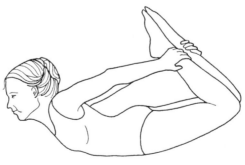

final position

Figure 13. The lower trunk stretcher

4. Pull with the belt or towel as you press back with the lower legs to make a small arch in the back.
5. Hold this position for ten to fifteen seconds the first day and gradually work up to one minute.
6. Breathe naturally while holding the position.

Intermediate Step 2: Using only the belt or towel, repeat the same procedure as before, but use more pressure with your arms and legs to arch the back without the cushions for the knees. Again, gradually work up to holding the position for one minute.

Final Position

1. Lie flat on your abdomen.
2. Bend the knees as fully as possible.
3. Reach back first with one hand and then with the other to grasp the ankles.
4. Keeping the arms straight and the head up, try to extend the knee joints, pressing the back into an arched position. Try to get your knees as high as possible.
5. Breathe naturally and hold the position for ten to fifteen seconds the first day, gradually increasing to one minute.
6. Release very slowly and gently.

Benefits: This position provides all the benefits of Exercise 1, and it strengthens and tones the lower back muscles and buttocks while stretching the hip flexors and the muscles on the front of the thighs.

Exercise 3:
The Upper Back Stretcher

The upper back stretcher is easy for most people, and it prepares you for Exercise 4.

1. Kneel on the floor with your toes pointed so that your weight is borne by the entire front of your shins and insteps, keeping the buttocks in contact with the calves.
2. Bend forward and try to place your head so that your scalp is on the floor, with your forehead in contact with your knees.
3. Stretch the arms forward until the elbows are straight and the palms of the hands are on the floor.
4. Hold the position for ten to fifteen seconds the first day and increase gradually to one minute. Maintain normal (slow, easy) breathing throughout.

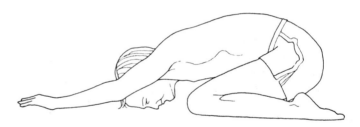

intermediate position

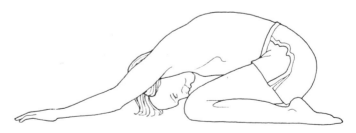

final position

Figure 14. The upper back stretcher

Intermediate Step: The only intermediate step needed to achieve the final position is allowing several inches between your head and knees. Continue to strive toward the final position.

Benefits: This position stretches the muscles and connective tissues of the upper back, particularly those of the cervical and thoracic regions. The extension of the arms overhead stretches the major muscles of the upper back.

Exercise 4:
The Upper and Lower Back Stretcher

Very few older people—especially older men—can do the upper and lower back stretches. Work toward the ultimate position only if it's easy for you. Figure 15 shows a more realistic goal for most older people. Even this may require months of persistent effort. Use the intermediate steps in order to progress.

Intermediate Step 1: You'll need a belt or small bath towel.

1. Sit on the floor with legs extended, knees locked, and feet together.
2. Loop the belt or towel around your feet.
3. Pulling on the belt with your hands, stretch to bring your head as close to your feet as possible without bending your knees. Don't bend your knees at any point! Use a longer belt rather than cheat by bending your knees, an action that changes the entire exercise anatomically.
4. Enter the position very gently. Do not, under any circumstances, bounce your body in this position.
5. Hold for a few seconds. Release very slowly and gently.
6. Repeat three times.

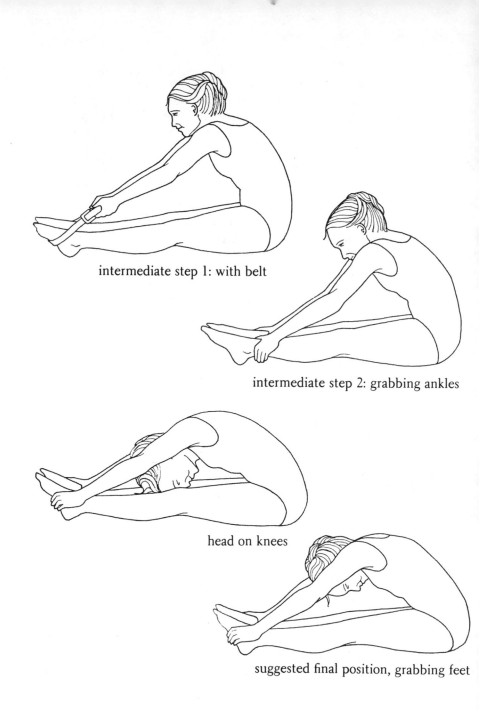

intermediate step 1: with belt

intermediate step 2: grabbing ankles

head on knees

suggested final position, grabbing feet

Figure 15. The upper and lower back stretcher

7. Over a period of days or weeks, work up to holding the position for one minute.

Intermediate Step 2: Follow the same steps and procedures as in the first intermediate step, but discard the belt and grasp your ankles.

Final Position: Repeat the first intermediate step, but grasp and hold the outer borders of the feet. The exceptionally flexible person will be able to rest the head on the knees while the elbows rest on the ground.

A word of caution: It is possible to trigger a spasm if you bounce your body while these muscles are stretched. Entering the position too vigorously is akin to bouncing. Be sure to enter and release the position very slowly. Never stretch beyond the point of mild discomfort. Pain is a sign that you're being overzealous.

Benefits: This exercise stretches every muscle in the back part of the body from head to toe. These muscles, often fatigued by poor posture, can be the site of small muscle spasms that bring about the excruciating pain of the low back syndrome. This stretching relaxes all these muscles and helps prevent muscle spasm.

Exercise 5:
The Neck Stretcher

The intermediate positions of the neck stretcher are not difficult, but the final position may be hard for many to achieve.

Intermediate Step 1: You'll need a footstool.

1. Lie flat on your back on the floor with the footstool about one to two feet from the top of your head.

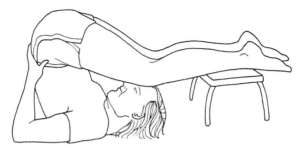

intermediate step 1: legs straight, feet on footstool, hands on hips

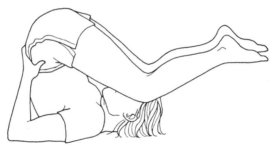

intermediate step 2: no footstool, legs bent at knees, hands on hips

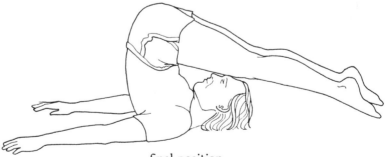

final position

Figure 16. The neck stretcher

2. Raise your legs over your head by bending the knees and then rolling up slowly, raising one vertebra off the floor at a time. Then straighten your knees and place the insteps and front of the legs on the footstool.
3. Support your hips with your hands, helping to keep the weight of your legs on the stool.
4. Hold for twenty to thirty seconds. Work up gradually to a minute.
5. Return to the original position by bringing your legs down with knees bent to prevent a heavy fall.

Intermediate Step 2: Repeat intermediate step 1 without the footstool. Allow more of the weight to come over your head by bending the knees. Work from twenty to thirty seconds up to a minute.

Final Position: Modify intermediate step 2 by placing your hands at your sides, palms down, at the start and leaving them in place as you press down with your hands to help get your legs overhead. The legs must remain straight, with the toes pointed. Progress from twenty to thirty seconds up to one minute.

Benefits: This position primarily stretches the muscles of the neck and the hamstrings, both frequent sites for stiffness, aches, and pains. Maintaining good mobility lessens such complaints and may provide complete relief.

Exercise 6:
The Trunk Twister

The final position of the trunk twister is difficult, but two relatively easy intermediate steps help you attain it.

Intermediate Step 1

1. Start in a sitting position with your legs straight and together.
2. Bring your right foot over your left knee and place it flat on the floor alongside your left knee.
3. Turn your head and shoulders slowly to the right as far as possible while grasping your left leg below the knee with your left hand.
4. Place your right hand on the floor behind you as far as possible to the left of your buttocks.
5. Hold the position, breathing normally, for ten to fifteen seconds the first day. Work toward a minute gradually.
6. Repeat in the opposite direction.

Intermediate Step 2

1. Start in the sitting position, as for intermediate step 1.
2. Bend your left knee as fully as possible without pain, so that the lower leg is folded against the thigh. If possible, your left heel should be under your right buttock, but this is not essential.
3. Bring your right foot over your left knee and place it flat on the floor alongside your left knee.
4. Reach across your right leg with your left arm to grasp your left knee with your left hand, with the back of your left arm resting on the outside of the right knee.
5. Turn your head and shoulders as far to the right as possible.
6. Place your right hand on the floor behind you as far as possible to the left of your buttocks.
7. Hold the position ten to fifteen seconds the first day, and gradually work toward one minute.
8. Repeat in the other direction.

Final Position

1. Start in the same sitting position as in the two intermediate steps.
2. Same as in intermediate step 2.
3. Same as in intermediate step 2.

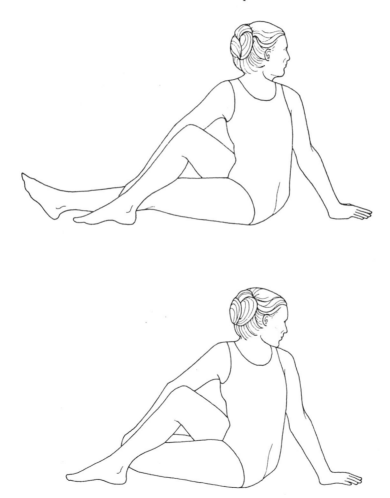

Figure 17. The trunk twister

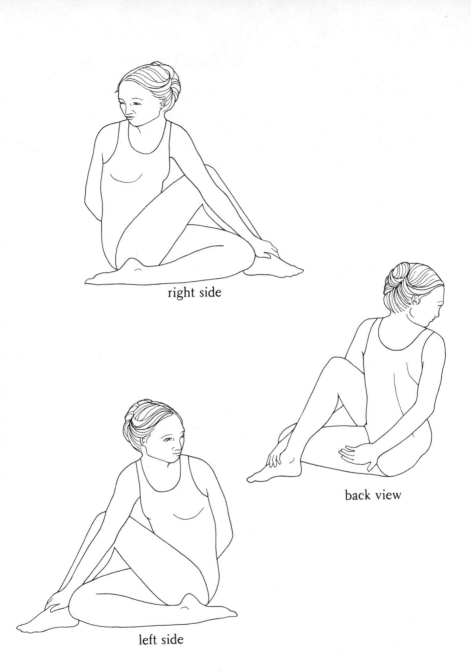

right side

back view

left side

Figure 17. The trunk twister (*Continued*)

4. Grasp the *ankle* of your right leg with your left hand (rather than grasping your left knee, as you did in intermediate step 2).
5. Turn your head and shoulders as far right as possible.
6. Bring your right hand around behind your back as far as possible to place your fingers, palm down, on your left thigh.
7. Hold for ten to fifteen seconds the first day, and gradually work toward one minute.
8. Repeat in the other direction.

Benefits: This exercise stretches the muscles of the trunk that do not run lengthwise. The lower part of the trunk and spine is locked in one direction, while the upper parts are rotated as far as possible in the opposite direction. This exercise keeps the muscles of the trunk, particularly those involved with spinal rotation, in good, supple condition. In turn, this helps produce good posture and the muscle balance essential to relieve backache.

Exercise 7:
The Toe Pointer

The toe pointer helps prevent or relieve shin splints. This exercise is not extremely difficult, but two intermediate positions will help the less flexible.

Intermediate Step 1

1. Kneel on the floor with feet together, toes extended behind.
2. Place your hands on the floor alongside your knees and rock your weight onto the insteps until you feel the pressure in the ankles and in the muscles on the front of the lower leg.

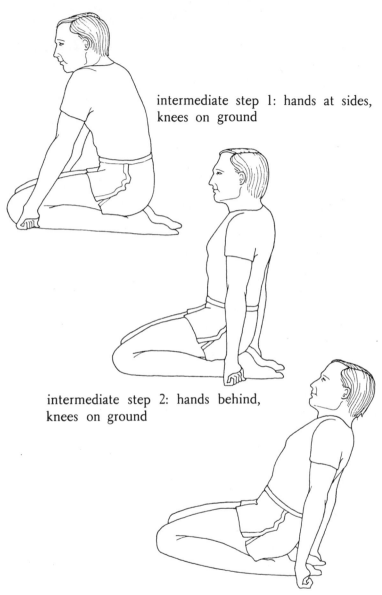

intermediate step 1: hands at sides, knees on ground

intermediate step 2: hands behind, knees on ground

final position: knees off floor

Figure 18. The toe pointer

3. Hold the position for ten to fifteen seconds, and work toward one minute.

Intermediate Step 2

1. Kneel on the floor, as in intermediate step 1, but place your hands on the floor behind you so you can catch your weight on your hands.
2. Rock your weight back so that most of your weight rests over your feet.
3. Hold for fifteen to twenty seconds, and work up to one minute.

Final Position

1. Kneel on the floor as in intermediate step 2, but rock your weight gently backward until it comes back far enough to bring your knees off the ground.
2. Hold for five to ten seconds, and gradually work up to one minute.

CAUTION: If you have or have had any knee problems, consult your physician before doing this exercise.

Benefits: This exercise prevents the pain many people develop in the front of the lower legs after vigorous walking or jogging. It also relieves these shin splints when they've already been brought about by excessive use of the lower legs.

Exercise 8:
The Calf and Shoulder Stretcher

You'll need a doorway with unobstructed wall space on each side.

1. Stand facing the doorway with your feet shoulder-width apart and about twelve inches from the doorway. Keep your feet pointed straight forward.
2. Extend your arms horizontally, straight at the elbow.
3. Lean forward slowly, resting your upper body weight on your arms against the walls, allowing your head and upper body to enter the doorway. Your weight will be resting on your forearms or upper arms, depending on your width and the width of the doorway.
4. Keep the arms straight at the elbows and make fists with your hands, keeping the backs of your hands pointing upward. Keep your knees and body straight throughout the exercise and your heels on the floor.
5. Hold for five to ten seconds the first day, and gradually work up to a minute.
6. To progress, place your feet farther and farther from the wall. When you can sustain a minute in position with your feet twelve inches from the doorway, attempt the same position from eighteen inches. Again, start at ten to fifteen seconds, and work up to a minute.

Benefits: A persistent soreness in the muscles of the calf is a common complaint after brisk walking or jogging if one is unused to such activity. This exercise prevents such soreness, improves the suppleness of the lower leg muscles and the elasticity of the connective tissue around the ankle joint, and helps relieve aches and pains in the shoulder. As we grow older, we use the arms and shoulder joints less and less throughout the full range of motion, and we tend to develop such pains and shrug them off as "bursitis." If you have such pains and they have been identified as true bursitis, consult your physician before doing this or the next exercise. If the aches are not due to bursitis, these exercises should relieve them.

Exercise 9:
The Shoulder and Biceps Stretcher

You'll need a dresser, a bookshelf, or some other piece of furniture whose top surface is at or only slightly below shoulder level.

1. Stand with your back to the dresser, about one foot away from it, with your feet shoulder-width apart.
2. Interlace your fingers behind your back, clasping your hands palm to palm.
3. Bend forward at the waist, allowing your arms to come up easily behind you, and place your clasped hands on the dresser top or shelf.
4. Straighten your body slowly and gently until you feel *mild* discomfort in your arms and/or shoulders.
5. Hold for five to ten seconds. Work toward a minute in this position.
6. To progress, stand more and more erect. If you are quite flexible, you may eventually need to raise the height of your hands by placing a book or two on the shelf or dresser top.

Benefits: This exercise provides a static stretch for the biceps muscles, which otherwise are very difficult to stretch. It also stretches part of the deltoid (shoulder) muscles, which often become painful as the result of unusual movements. Together with Exercise 8, this stretch relieves minor but annoying shoulder pains, a common complaint of older persons.

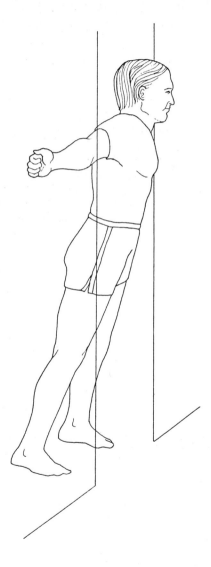

Figure 19. The calf and shoulder stretcher

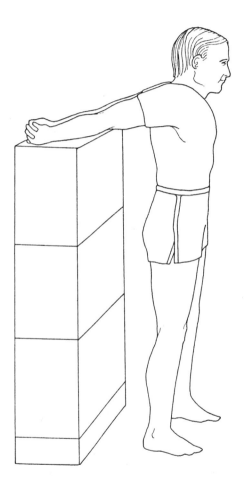

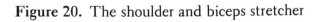

Figure 20. The shoulder and biceps stretcher

RETESTING

After six weeks at Level One, retest yourself on the PPR test to observe your progress. If you're above average on all four stepping rates, you're ready for Level Two, even though you might not have completed the entire progressive walking program. If you score at least in the average category on all four stepping rates and complete the entire progressive walking program without exceeding the heart rate limit of 120 beats per minute, you also may advance to Level Two.

If you don't meet either of these criteria (or if your physician wants you to remain at Level One), continue at Level One for six more weeks. Don't be impatient. Even the Level One program brings about significant improvements in fitness for men and women over 50.

10

Exercises:
Level Two

At Level Two, as at Level One, each workout consists of three parts. The first is a jog-walk program (instead of the progressive walking used at Level One). In the second part, you perform the same calisthenics as in Level One, except that you do more repetitions in each two-minute period. Static stretching—the third part—remains the same. No advancements beyond the final positions described in the preceding chapter are necessary, but you should work to hold these positions for a full minute. Once you reach that goal, you should continue the stretching as the final cooling-down phase of every workout.

THE JOG-WALK PROGRAM

The goal of the jog-walk program is to improve your heart, lungs, and muscles to the point where you can jog one mile, without stopping, easily and without strain. You progress toward this goal by alternating a given number of steps jogged with a given number of steps walked. You set your own rate—the chief determinant of the exercise's stressfulness—at a level comfortable for you.

How is jogging different from running? Running implies speed, and in this program we are not interested in speed. We define jogging as a slow trot, the first step up from walking toward running. Because jogging is more like walking than running, form is not so important. However, we're offering a few pointers to improve your efficiency in jogging and prevent unnecessary problems.

Posture matters. Jog with your head up and body erect, or else you won't be able to expand the lungs fully.

Stay loose. Don't tense up or force yourself in any way. Jogging must be done easily, naturally, and without strain.

Keep all movements in the forward-backward direction; any crosswise movements would be literally at cross-purposes to your goal. Point your feet straight ahead. (You can check whether you're doing this by observing your footprints on sand or soft ground or on pavement after jogging through a puddle.) Let your arms swing easily in rhythm with your leg motion—not across your body, but forward and backward. The way the foot strikes the ground varies from person to person. Speed runners run on the ball of the foot. In jogging, most people find it most natural to bring the whole foot into contact with the ground with each step. Bringing the foot down heel first suits most people best. However, you may prefer to touch down with the ball of the foot. Do whatever comes naturally for you.

Buy good-quality running shoes with thick, resilient soles. They should fit a bit more snugly than street shoes so that your feet cannot slip or slide within them. If the eyelets for the laces come closer to each other than about one inch, the shoes probably are cut too wide for your foot. Select another brand that's cut better for you. Of course, don't get shoes that are too tight for comfort. You probably can get more reliable information and assistance from a sales clerk in a sporting goods store than from one in a general department store or shoe store.

Breathe through both the nose and the mouth to get enough oxygen. Unlike the other exercises, which require only regular breathing, jogging demands more oxygen than your nose alone can provide. It is this challenge to your respiratory system that deepens and expands your breathing capacity.

Consider the weather. In regions where winter is long and hard, you may have to change when and what you do. Sometimes just changing your schedule is enough. For example, after a week of cold, icy weather that made jogging impossible and kept you indoors, you could make it up by walking every day for a week until you can get back on schedule. Alternatively, during the cold spell you could combine walking up and down a hallway with jogging in place. This substitute isn't quite so strenuous as the real jog-walk program, but it won't seriously affect your training.

Another possibility is to use stool-stepping at a rate and duration roughly equivalent to the point you have reached in the jog-walk program. To do this, look at your most recent PPR test results and select the rate of stool-stepping that evokes the heart rate response most similar to that recorded for your last day's jog-walk. Do this by dividing the two-minute recovery pulse rate of the test by two and adding twenty beats per minute to the result. This is a rough approximation of your heart rate during stepping. Fifty steps of jogging take approximately twenty seconds, so do the stool-stepping for twenty seconds. Take your heart rate and walk the appropriate number of steps for your walk interval. At the end of your walk, you should be back at the stepping stool again.

Another possible substitution is rope skipping, but it is recommended only if you have some skill at it. And it must be done by trial and error until you establish the heart rate response to various paces and methods of rope skipping.

The Game Plan

You start the jog-walk program with a very modest challenge to your cardiovascular and respiratory systems. First you'll modify the distance jogged. Later you'll modify the intensity by shortening the walking or rest periods. This "double-progressive" training procedure has been proven effective for persons over 50 both in laboratory experiments and in practical experience.

Every day you perform from five to ten sets of jog-walking. Each set consists of a given number of steps jogged and a given number of steps walked during the "rest" interval. The first day you do five sets of fifty steps jogging and fifty steps walking. The second day you do six sets, the third day seven, and so on until you've completed ten sets of fifty steps jogging and fifty steps walking. You progress to this point only by increasing your duration or distance, which increases the demands on your heart and lungs very gently.

Once you've completed ten of these sets, you're ready to increase the intensity of your exercise in either of two ways: by moving faster or by cutting down the rest (walking) interval. The latter is safer: You jog fifty steps and walk only forty, but you do only five sets of this new plan. (See Table 3, page 129.)

If you're in your fifties or sixties, set yourself a heart rate limit of 140 beats per minute throughout the program. If you are 70 or older, your limit is 130 beats. These levels mean that you're staying below 85 percent of your maximum, a very effective level for training a healthy older person without danger of overstress.

Take your heart rate immediately after each fifty-step jog interval. As long as it stays under your limit, follow the progression outlined in Table 3. If you go over your limit, you may be jogging too fast. If not, increase the walk interval by ten steps and then return to the appropriate point of progression.

If you train three times a week at an average rate of progress, you'll arrive at the "individual program," the final goal, in about six months. The next step is jogging steadily for a quarter-mile, checking your heart rate at the end. If it's under the limit, you may increase your jogging distance by an eighth of a mile until you reach the ultimate goal of one mile of continuous jogging without rest *and* without exceeding the heart rate limit.

After completing the sets of the jog-walk or continuous jogging, be sure to walk for an additional two or three minutes to cool down your body gradually.

When you first complete a mile of jogging, your time for that distance may vary between nine and twelve minutes, depending on your age and your lifetime history of physical activity. Some older men who have run marathons do far better than nine minutes for a mile, but a faster speed isn't necessary for optimal levels of health and physical fitness. If you're competitive and want to shoot for maximum performance, consult your physician again before you attempt any pace faster than a nine-minute mile.

Off and Running

You'll need some equipment for the jog-walk: your stopwatch or wristwatch with sweep-second hand, a small clipboard, a pencil, and your copy of Chart 3 on page 140. If you can or must walk to and from a jogging course, so much the better.

Jogging itself is an excellent warm-up, so start out with fifty steps jogging. Stop and take your pulse. Eventually you'll be able to measure your heart rate without stopping completely; you'll test your pulse during the walking interval. On the first day, start your fifty steps of walking as soon as you've measured your heart rate. Then start the next fifty steps of jogging. Record your heart rate after each of the five jogging sessions. It is important that you take your heart rate as quickly as possible after the jog interval.

If you exceed your heart rate limit on the first day, add ten steps to the walk period. On the second day you would then take fifty jogging steps and sixty walking steps. If at any point you consistently hit the heart rate limit, spend an extra day or several days at the same step without progressing. Remember that time is not the point. The important factor is your circulatory system's ability to respond to the challenge of exercise without undue stress.

Table 4 gives the estimated heart rate responses to various levels of jog-walking according to physical fitness level. It's designed to determine the appropriate starting level of jog-walk for those who found the fifty jog–fifty walk program too easy on the first day, as indicated by a heart rate considerably below 130, and for those who scored "excellent" or "very good" on the progressive pulse rate test.

If you determine that you should start the jog-walk program at a level higher than fifty jog steps and fifty walk steps, the same general instructions and plan of progression still apply to you. The only difference is the starting point. Do five sets at the appropriate level on the first day, and progress from there.

CALISTHENICS

Your muscular strength, endurance, and flexibility do not necessarily improve at the same rate as your circulatory-respiratory responses to walking and the jog-walk. Even if you're ready for Level Two in jogging, you must not advance into the second level of calisthenics until you can easily achieve, without exceeding a heart rate limit of 120 beats, the following repetitions of the calisthenics:

1. Bender: 20 in two minutes
2. Easy push-up: 40 in two minutes
3. Slow-motion flutter kick: 20 in two minutes
4. Easy sit-up: 40 in two minutes

If you can attain these goals, you're ready for Level Two of the calisthenics program.

Exercise 1:
The Bender

Continue the bender just as in Level One (see page 82), but gradually increase your rate toward a maximum of forty in two minutes.

Exercise 2:
The Full Body Push-up (for Men Only)

The full body push-up is a two-count exercise. The starting position and counting are the same as for the easy push-up (see page 83). The only difference is that when you push up, the body remains straight from feet to shoulders, creating more resistance. Resist any temptation to do this exercise to the point of straining. And don't hold your breath. At the first sign of difficulty, lower your body gently down to the floor and rest. This exercise is usually advisable only for men in very good shape. Women and most men should continue doing the easy push-up.

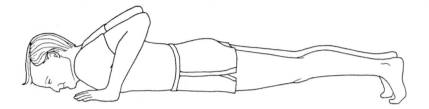

count one

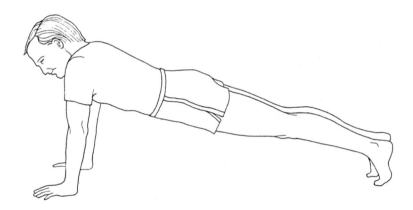

count two

Figure 21. The full body push-up

Exercise 3:
The Flutter Kick

The Level Two flutter kick is like the slow-motion flutter kick of Level One (see page 85), but now you increase the cadence to a maximum of forty in a two-minute period.

Exercise 4:
The Full Body Sit-up

The full body sit-up is a two-count exercise. Start flat on your back with hands behind your neck and knees bent (see Fig. 22, page 120). You may lock your feet under a piece of furniture or have a partner hold them for you.

Count 1: Lift your head, shoulders, and upper body off the floor and bring the right elbow forward to touch the left knee.

Count 2: Return to starting position. Alternate with left elbow to right knee.

You may gradually increase the cadence up to twenty per minute for a total of forty sit-ups. However, this is neither desirable nor necessary.

STATIC STRETCHING

The static stretching exercises remain the same in Level Two as in Level One. The ultimate goal is to achieve the final positions and hold them for one minute.

You'll notice that the Level Two program is shorter than Level One: thirty to forty-five minutes rather than an hour. This is time and exercise enough to maintain your physical fitness for the rest of your life, if you repeat the program three to five times a week.

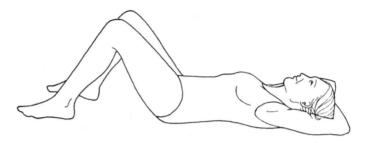

count one

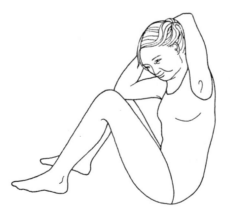

count two

Figure 22. The full body sit-up

11

Fitness for Life

We have said that the exercise prescription given in this book is an approach to fitness for persons over 50 that has been proven both safe and effective. Of course, we cannot and do not claim that it is the only way to achieve fitness. Many types of exercises improve the function of the circulatory and respiratory systems: swimming, tennis, bicycling, handball, squash, and others. We did not include these because our program requires activities that can be measured in a controlled, quantitative way and that can be adjusted for intensity, duration, and frequency. We had to be scientific in determining the appropriate dose-response for the unconditioned older man or woman.

We also were wary of the liabilities of other activities. Take swimming as an example. For a skilled person, this is one of the finest exercises. However, only a small percentage of older men and women have the high skill level required to swim far enough and long enough to benefit the heart, lungs, and circulation. There is also the problem of finding a suitable, affordable, uncrowded year-round facility. Moreover, swimming may be unsuitable for some people because of residual medical problems, such as sinusitis or a tendency to ear infections. Another fine conditioner is bicycling, but it can be hazardous in cities and impossible during long winters.

Progressive walking and the jog-walk program, by comparison, meet the needs of the greatest number of people. These activities, done according to this program, are safe and effective and involve minimal cost for equipment. If, after you've achieved a high level of fitness, you wish to return to a sport that you used to enjoy, go ahead. This program will have given you the ability to monitor your safety and progress by measuring your heart rate and by learning how to stay within certain heart rate limits. The progressive pulse rate test can be used to assess your progress on any form of conditioning.

If you do wish to add a sport to your fitness plan, here are some recommendations:

1. Clear the proposed sports program with your doctor.
2. Follow the basic fitness program two days a week.
3. If your chosen sport is very vigorous, don't add more than two days a week. Don't add more than three days of sports activity of any sort.
4. Check your heart rate frequently in the early stages of the added program.
5. Perform the static stretching exercises after the sports activity to prevent muscle soreness and to maintain mobility.
6. Check your fitness level with the progressive pulse rate test monthly for the first six months of the new activity. Any drop in your score is a

probable indication that you are overdoing it. In this case, reduce the new activity to one day per week and continue the standard Level Two program two days a week.

Bear in mind that the exercise prescription in this book is not a one-time cure-all. Even though you will see dramatic improvements in just a few weeks, think in terms of the long haul—of months, years, and decades of fitness. Unlike the quick-weight-loss, inches-off-in-seven-days schemes that you find in the tabloids, this plan is designed to provide long-term benefits.

At no point does the fitness program demand a great deal of your time and energy. Our volunteers exercise three hours a week—three of the 112 or so waking hours of the average person. And the exercise sessions have definite limits on exertion as well as time. The payoff on these relatively small investments of energy and time is long-term and high: lower blood pressure, more energy, less tension, greater flexibility, and a sense of positive well-being.

The key to these dividends is *regular* exercise sessions. You may have tried other diets or exercise plans in the past and quit because they asked too much of your self-restraint or your muscles. Take it slow on this program. Gradually add these activities to your daily habits until they become part of your routine. And don't work toward a goal and quit when you reach it. Fitness demands continued workouts. Staying fit requires less effort than becoming fit, but you can't make that effort in bits and spurts. We recommend a minimum of three workouts a week.

Doing too much can be as much of a hazard as doing too little. This is a noncompetitive program. Speed is not of the essence. There's no incentive for rushing through the plan and trying to do more in less time than anyone else. The level of exertion has been chosen because it is the ideal for gaining maximum benefits with maximum safety. Doing more won't bring more improvements— and it could reverse some of the progress you have made.

The best measure of the value of this program is the improvement you will observe in your own health and vigor as you progress with the exercises. We aren't saying that these activities will bring you back to the way you were in your teens, but they will help you to trim off fat, firm up your muscles, and infuse new energy into your work and play. Over time, this program can make you look better and feel healthier. And with regular exercise, you can keep up this level of fitness for many years to come.

Appendix 1:

Heart Rate Conversion Tables

Table A. Conversion of Time for 20 Beats to Heart Rate (Beats per Minute)

Time	Heart Rate	Time	Heart Rate	Time	Heart Rate	Time	Heart Rate
20.0	60	18.6	65	17.2	70	15.8	76
19.9	60	18.5	65	17.1	70	15.7	76
19.8	61	18.4	65	17.0	71	15.6	77
19.7	61	18.3	66	16.9	71	15.5	77
19.6	61	18.2	66	16.8	71	15.4	78
19.5	62	18.1	66	16.7	72	15.3	78
19.4	62	18.0	67	16.6	72	15.2	79
19.3	62	17.9	67	16.5	73	15.1	79
19.2	63	17.8	67	16.4	73	15.0	80
19.1	63	17.7	68	16.3	74	14.9	81
19.0	63	17.6	68	16.2	74	14.8	81
18.9	63	17.5	69	16.1	75	14.7	82
18.8	64	17.4	69	16.0	75	14.6	82
18.7	64	17.3	69	15.9	75	14.5	83

Table A. Conversion of Time for 20 Beats to Heart Rate
(Beats per Minute) (*Continued*)

Time	Heart Rate	Time	Heart Rate	Time	Heart Rate	Time	Heart Rate
14.4	83	12.1	99	9.8	122	7.5	160
14.3	84	12.0	100	9.7	124	7.4	162
14.2	85	11.9	101	9.6	125	7.3	164
14.1	85	11.8	102	9.5	126	7.2	167
14.0	86	11.7	103	9.4	128	7.1	169
13.9	86	11.6	103	9.3	129	7.0	171
13.8	87	11.5	104	9.2	130	6.9	174
13.7	88	11.4	105	9.1	132	6.8	176
13.6	88	11.3	106	9.0	133	6.7	179
13.5	89	11.2	107	8.9	135	6.6	182
13.4	89	11.1	108	8.8	136	6.5	185
13.3	90	11.0	109	8.7	138	6.4	188
13.2	91	10.9	110	8.6	140	6.3	190
13.1	92	10.8	111	8.5	141	6.2	194
13.0	92	10.7	112	8.4	143	6.1	197
12.9	93	10.6	113	8.3	145	6.0	200
12.8	94	10.5	114	8.2	146	5.9	203
12.7	94	10.4	115	8.1	148	5.8	207
12.6	95	10.3	116	8.0	150	5.7	211
12.5	96	10.2	117	7.9	152	5.6	214
12.4	97	10.1	118	7.8	154	5.5	218
12.3	98	10.0	120	7.7	156		
12.2	98	9.9	121	7.6	158		

Table B. Conversion of Beats Counted in 10 Seconds to Heart Rate (Beats per Minute)

Beats in 10 seconds	Heart Rate
10	60
11	66
12	72
13	78
14	84
15	90
16	96
17	102
18	108
19	114
20	120
21	126
22	132
23	138
24	144
25	150
26	156
27	162
28	168
29	174

Appendix 2:

Personal Record Charts

Table 1. Progressive Walking Program

Workout Day	Distance (miles)	Time (minutes)	Rate
1	1	20	
2	1¼	25	
3	1½	30	
4	1¾	35	
5	2	40	20 min. per mile
6	2¼	45	
7	2½	50	
8	2¾	55	
9	3	60	
10	2	32	
11	2¼	36	
12	2½	40	
13	2¾	44	
14	3	48	16 min. per mile
15	3¼	52	
16	3½	56	
17	3¾	60	
18	4	64	

Table 2. Level One Calisthenics

Exercises	Rate	Time (minutes)	Repetitions
1. Bender	4 per min.	2	8
2. Easy push-up	5 per min.	2	10
3. Slow-motion flutter kick	8 per min.	2	16
4. Easy sit-up	8 per min.	2	16

Table 3. Jog-Walk Program

Days	Jog	Walk	Number of Sets*
1 → 6	50 steps	50 steps	5 → 10
7 → 12	50 steps	40 steps	5 → 10
13 → 18	50 steps	30 steps	5 → 10
19 → 24	50 steps	20 steps	5 → 10
25 → 30	50 steps	10 steps	5 → 10
31 → 36	75 steps	10 steps	5 → 10
37 → 42	100 steps	10 steps	5 → 10
43 → 48	125 steps	10 steps	5 → 10
49 → 54	150 steps	10 steps	5 → 10
55 → 60	175 steps	10 steps	5 → 10
61 → 66	200 steps	10 steps	5 → 10
67 →	Individualized program		

*Increase number of sets by one each day at each level of exercise.

Table 4. Maximum Heart Rate in Five Sets of Jog-Walking*

Fitness category (PPR test)	50 jog steps 50 walk steps	50 jog steps 40 walk steps	50 jog steps 30 walk steps	50 jog steps 20 walk steps	50 jog steps 10 walk steps
Excellent	110 (102–118)	115 (107–123)	119 (111–127)	122 (114–130)	126 (118–134)
Very good	113 (105–121)	118 (110–126)	122 (114–130)	124 (116–132)	128 (120–136)
Average	117 (109–125)	122 (114–130)	125 (117–133)	128 (120–136)	133 (125–141)
Below average	122 (114–130)	126 (118–134)	130 (122–138)	132 (124–140)	137 (129–145)
Poor	126 (118–134)	128 (120–136)	132 (124–140)	135 (127–143)	140 (132–148)

*These data were established in Dr. H. A. deVries's laboratory by radiotelemetry methods. The upper figure represents the average heart rate response. The lower figures represent the range for plus or minus one standard deviation.

Table 5. Level Two Calisthenics

Exercises	Rate	Time (minutes)	Repetitions
1. Bender	10–20 per min.	2	20–40
2. Full body push-up	as you please		as many as possible without strain
3. Flutter kick	10–20 per min.	2	20–40
4. Full body sit-up	10–20 per min.	2	20–40

Chart 1.* Progressive Pulse Rate Test: Before Conditioning

	Total 2-Minute Pulse Count			
Classification	after 12 4-step cycles per min.	after 18 4-step cycles per min.	after 21 4-step cycles per min.	after 30 4-step cycles per min.
Excellent	102	110	114	125
	106	114	118	130
	110	118	122	135
	114	122	126	140
	118	126	130	145
Above average	122	130	134	150
	126	134	138	155
	130	138	142	160
	134	142	146	165
	138	146	150	170
Average	142	150	154	175
	146	154	158	180
	150	158	162	185
	154	162	166	190
	158	166	170	195
Below average	162	170	174	200
	166	174	178	205
	170	178	182	210
	174	182	186	215
	178	186	190	220
Poor	182	190	194	225
	186	194	198	230
	190	198	202	235
	194	202	206	240
	198	206	210	245

*Data compiled by Dr. H. A. deVries, K. S. Ambe, and G. M. Adams.

Progressive Pulse Rate Test:
After 6 Weeks of Conditioning

	Total 2-Minute Pulse Count			
Classification	after 12 4-step cycles per min.	after 18 4-step cycles per min.	after 24 4-step cycles per min.	after 30 4-step cycles per min.
	102	110	114	125
	106	114	118	130
Excellent	110	118	122	135
	114	122	126	140
	118	126	130	145
	122	130	134	150
	126	134	138	155
Above average	130	138	142	160
	134	142	146	165
	138	146	150	170
	142	150	154	175
	146	154	158	180
Average	150	158	162	185
	154	162	166	190
	158	166	170	195
	162	170	174	200
	166	174	178	205
Below average	170	178	182	210
	174	182	186	215
	178	186	190	220
	182	190	194	225
	186	194	198	230
Poor	190	198	202	235
	194	202	206	240
	198	206	210	245

Progressive Pulse Rate Test:
After 12 Weeks of Conditioning

Classification	Total 2-Minute Pulse Count			
	after 12 4-step cycles per min.	after 18 4-step cycles per min.	after 24 4-step cycles per min.	after 30 4-step cycles per min.
Excellent	102	110	114	125
	106	114	118	130
	110	118	122	135
	114	122	126	140
	118	126	130	145
Above average	122	130	134	150
	126	134	138	155
	130	138	142	160
	134	142	146	165
	138	146	150	170
Average	142	150	154	175
	146	154	158	180
	150	158	162	185
	154	162	166	190
	158	166	170	195
Below average	162	170	174	200
	166	174	178	205
	170	178	182	210
	174	182	186	215
	178	186	190	220
Poor	182	190	194	225
	186	194	198	230
	190	198	202	235
	194	202	206	240
	198	206	210	245

Progressive Pulse Rate Test:
After 24 Weeks of Conditioning

Classification	Total 2-Minute Pulse Count			
	after 12 4-step cycles per min.	after 18 4-step cycles per min.	after 24 4-step cycles per min.	after 30 4-step cycles per min.
Excellent	102	110	114	125
	106	114	118	130
	110	118	122	135
	114	122	126	140
	118	126	130	145
Above average	122	130	134	150
	126	134	138	155
	130	138	142	160
	134	142	146	165
	138	146	150	170
Average	142	150	154	175
	146	154	158	180
	150	158	162	185
	154	162	166	190
	158	166	170	195
Below average	162	170	174	200
	166	174	178	205
	170	178	182	210
	174	182	186	215
	178	186	190	220
Poor	182	190	194	225
	186	194	198	230
	190	198	202	235
	194	202	206	240
	198	206	210	245

Progressive Pulse Rate Test:
After 1 Year of Conditioning

	Total 2-Minute Pulse Count			
Classification	after 12 4-step cycles per min.	after 18 4-step cycles per min.	after 24 4-step cycles per min.	after 30 4-step cycles per min.
Excellent	102	110	114	125
	106	114	118	130
	110	118	122	135
	114	122	126	140
	118	126	130	145
Above average	122	130	134	150
	126	134	138	155
	130	138	142	160
	134	142	146	165
	138	146	150	170
Average	142	150	154	175
	146	154	158	180
	150	158	162	185
	154	162	166	190
	158	166	170	195
Below average	162	170	174	200
	166	174	178	205
	170	178	182	210
	174	182	186	215
	178	186	190	220
Poor	182	190	194	225
	186	194	198	230
	190	198	202	235
	194	202	206	240
	198	206	210	245

Chart 2. Progress in Progressive Walking Program: First 6 Weeks

Name _____ Age _____ Resting Heart Rate (HR) _____

Exercise Progression	Date	HR	Date	HR	Date	HR	Date	HR
1. Walk 1 mile in 20 min.								
2. Walk 1¼ miles 25 min.								
3. Walk 1½ miles 30 min.								
4. Walk 1¾ miles 35 min.								
5. Walk 2 miles 40 min.								
6. Walk 2¼ miles 45 min.								
7. Walk 2½ miles 50 min.								
8. Walk 2¾ miles 55 min.								

Exercise Progression	Date	HR	Date	HR	Date	HR	Date	HR	Date	HR
9. Walk 3 miles 1 hour										
10. Walk 2 miles 32 min.										
11. Walk 2¼ miles 36 min.										
12. Walk 2½ miles 40 min.										
13. Walk 2¾ miles 44 min.										
14. Walk 3 miles 48 min.										
15. Walk 3¼ miles 52 min.										
16. Walk 3½ miles 56 min.										
17. Walk 3¾ miles 1 hour										
18. Walk 4 miles 1 hour 4 min.										

137

Progress in Progressive Walking Program: Second 6 Weeks

Name _____ Age _____ Resting Heart Rate (HR) _____

Exercise Progression	Date	HR	Date	HR	Date	HR	Date	HR
1. Walk 1 mile in 20 min.								
2. Walk 1¼ miles 25 min.								
3. Walk 1½ miles 30 min.								
4. Walk 1¾ miles 30 min.								
5. Walk 2 miles 40 min.								
6. Walk 2¼ miles 45 min.								
7. Walk 2½ miles 50 min.								
8. Walk 2¾ miles 55 min.								
9. Walk 3 miles 1 hour								

Exercise Progression	Date	HR	Date	HR	Date	HR	Date	HR
10. Walk 2 miles 32 min.								
11. Walk 2¼ miles 36 min.								
12. Walk 2½ miles 40 min.								
13. Walk 2¾ miles 44 min.								
14. Walk 3 miles 48 min.								
15. Walk 3¼ miles 52 min.								
16. Walk 3½ miles 56 min.								
17. Walk 3¾ miles 1 hour								
18. Walk 4 miles 1 hour 4 min.								

Chart 3. Progress in Jog-Walk Program: First 6 Weeks

Name _____ Age ____ Resting Heart Rate (HR) ____

Date																				
1. No. of steps in jog interval																				
2. No. of steps in walk interval																				
3. No. of steps of jog-walk																				
4. HR at end of 1st jog																				
5. HR at end of 2nd jog																				
6. HR at end of 3rd jog																				
7. HR at end of 4th jog																				
8. HR at end of 5th jog																				
9. HR at end of 6th jog																				
10. HR at end of 7th jog																				
11. HR at end of 8th jog																				
12. HR at end of 9th jog																				
13. HR at end of 10th jog																				

Progress in Jog-Walk Program: Second 6 Weeks

Name _____ Age ____ ____ Resting Heart Rate (HR) ____

Date																			
1. No. of steps in jog interval																			
2. No. of steps in walk interval																			
3. No. of sets of jog-walk																			
4. HR at end of 1st jog																			
5. HR at end of 2nd jog																			
6. HR at end of 3rd jog																			
7. HR at end of 4th jog																			
8. HR at end of 5th jog																			
9. HR at end of 6th jog																			
10. HR at end of 7th jog																			
11. HR at end of 8th jog																			
12. HR at end of 9th jog																			
13. HR at end of 10th jog																			

Progress in Jog-Walk Program: Third 6 Weeks

Name _____ Age _____ Resting Heart Rate (HR) _____

Date																	
1. No. of steps in jog interval																	
2. No. of steps in walk interval																	
3. No. of sets of jog-walk																	
4. HR at end of 1st jog																	
5. HR at end of 2nd jog																	
6. HR at end of 3rd jog																	
7. HR at end of 4th jog																	
8. HR at end of 5th jog																	
9. HR at end of 6th jog																	
10. HR at end of 7th jog																	
11. HR at end of 8th jog																	
12. HR at end of 9th jog																	
13. HR at end of 10th jog																	

Progress in Jog-Walk Program: Fourth 6 Weeks

Name —————————— Age ——— Resting Heart Rate (HR) ———

Date																				
1. No. of steps in jog interval																				
2. No. of steps in walk interval																				
3. No. of sets of jog-walk																				
4. HR at end of 1st jog																				
5. HR at end of 2nd jog																				
6. HR at end of 3rd jog																				
7. HR at end of 4th jog																				
8. HR at end of 5th jog																				
9. HR at end of 6th jog																				
10. HR at end of 7th jog																				
11. HR at end of 8th jog																				
12. HR at end of 9th jog																				
13. HR at end of 10th jog																				

INDEX

Index